Healthcare Databases

A simple guide to building and using them

Alan Gillies

Professor in Information Management

University of Central Lancashire

Radcliffe Medical Press

Radcliffe Medical Press Ltd
18 Marcham Road
Abingdon
Oxon OX14 1AA
United Kingdom

www.radcliffe-oxford.com
The Radcliffe Medical Press electronic catalogue and online ordering facility.
Direct sales to anywhere in the world.

—————————————————————————————

British Library Cataloguing in Publication Data

A catalogue record for this book is available from the British Library.

ISBN 1 85775 972 9

Typeset by Joshua Associates Ltd, Oxford
Printed and bound by TJ International Ltd, Padstow, Cornwall

Contents

Preface

Who is this book for?

This book is for healthcare workers who really don't fancy all this technology. It is not for absolute beginners. For that, try *Excel for Clinical Governance* (another of my books, and currently my best seller). It assumes that you can use Windows, a mouse and know what a menu is (a collection of delicious food? Wrong answer – go to *Excel for Clinical Governance*, do not pass GO, do not collect £200).

However, it is intended to be readable, approachable and not to assume prior knowledge of databases. A typical reader might be one of the following.

- You have completed early modules of the ECDL and are now looking at the databases module and want a bit of help.
- You have completed all the ECDL and want to see how to apply it in a clinical context.
- You think that ECDL stands for Every Computer Deserves Lashing (actually it's the European Computer Driving Licence and the NHS is adopting it as a base IT qualification (-ish!)) but want to use a database to help you with a small audit/research project. You should ignore the 'ECDL' section of this preface!
- You're a clinician and you're fed up with not understanding a word that your daughters/IT people tell you
- You're a student of ours and need help with the practical work on the technology module.

Whoever you are, if you've got this far, welcome and please read on . . .

What will I need?

You will need access to a PC, with Microsoft Access 2000 or later. I have used Access 2000 as it's as recent a version as many people in the NHS will have. If you have Access XP, then I trust you will not find it a problem and enjoy the enhancements of the newer version.

There are some online resources to be found at the book's accompanying website **www.radcliffe-oxford.com/healthcaredatabases**. However, these are not quite an essential part of the book, so Internet or NHSnet access is desirable, but not essential.

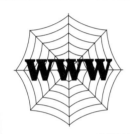

Web link
From the website accompanying this book you can download a range of useful but not quite essential items.

Features of the book

One of the main distinctive features of the book is **Smart Alec**:

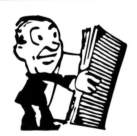

Smart Alec says
'Let me introduce myself. My name is Smart Alec and I am his (the author's) *alter ego*. I pop up throughout the text and throw in the asides that he would if he was teaching. Sometimes I just heckle him to keep up the interest level. It is alleged that some of you may find my presence irritating at times; if so, just ignore me, and I'll return the compliment. And despite rumours to the contrary, I do not wear an anorak.'

Another key feature are the **Over to you** sections:

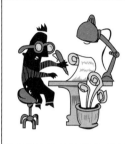

Over to you
These sections cover practical activities for you to do. In the first chapter they are conceptual in nature. In later chapters, where we are dealing with constructing a database application, they are tasks where you have already worked through a very similar task in the main text. They serve to reinforce and to build up confidence.

Finally, as you work though the text you will build up a model application. This is meant to help you understand what on earth is going on!

As you gain more confidence, the explanations do become a little sparser. If you find yourself getting a little lost, try slowing down a bit. Similarly, if you find the explanations becoming wearisome, then go and talk to my *alter ego*!

ECDL

In the table below, I have shown how the learning outcomes of ECDL are covered within this book.

	ECDL knowledge area	Covered in chapter	Notes
5.1	Getting started	Assumed knowledge	Covered in *Excel for Clinical Governance*, which also covers spreadsheets in greater detail than ECDL requires for module 4
5.2	Create a database	Chapter 2	
5.3	Use of forms	Chapter 3	
5.4	Retrieve information	Chapter 4	
5.5	Reporting	Chapter 4	Additional material provided on mail merging with Access: links to ECDL module 3

This book also provides an introduction to the theory of databases and sets the learning outcomes in a clinical context.

When I started this book it was meant to cover a range of key technology issues, including databases as well as Internet and networking issues. However, the scope of such a book became too large for one project, and it occurred to me that some people might not need the Internet bit and others might not need the databases bit. So it is intended that there will be a sequel to this book, not concerned with 'Even more Access', or, as I prefer to think of it, 'Access for Anoraks', but rather to deal with networks, the Internet and online data sources. However, it was intended that Channel tunnel trains would run direct from Manchester to Brussels, so the best laid plans . . .

Alan Gillies
professor@alangillies.com
June 2002

For Rachael

1

Designing a database

Introduction: what information do I need?

The starting point for any database is thinking about the information that you use and what you use it for.

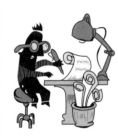

Over to you
To start us off, let's think about three relatively simple processes:

- as the receptionist, you take a phone call to book an appointment
- as the doctor, you receive a discharge letter from the hospital
- as the practice nurse, you give a set of travel injections.

Exercise 1.1 Information needs (1)

	Information item	*Purpose(s) for which that information is collected*
Phone call to book an appointment		

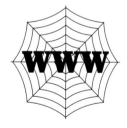

Web link

From the Chapter 1 section of the website accompanying this book you can download an Acrobat table template for you to print out and fill in.

Exercise 1.1 Information needs (2)

	Information item	Purpose(s) for which that information is collected
Receive discharge letter from hospital		

Exercise 1.1   Information needs (3)

	Information item	*Purpose(s) for which that information is collected*
Give a set of travel injections		

The task of writing a database to cover even this small part of the information needs is surprisingly complex.

Real world information needs in primary care

The information needs of any organisation should reflect the purpose of the organisation. You'd be amazed how often it's the other way around. This doesn't mean that when you put in a new computer system you don't change the way that you work: but it does mean that any changes should be made because the computer gives you the chance to work better or smarter, not just because the computer has limitations that it wants to impose on you!

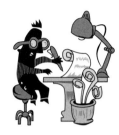

Over to you
Now try to identify the three most important objectives of your practice. Identify key tasks needed to achieve them and the key pieces of information you need to support these activities.

Exercise 1.2 Supporting key objectives

Key practice objective	Activities needed to achieve this objective	Information needed to support this activity

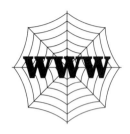

Web link
From the Chapter 1 section of the website accompanying this book you can download an Acrobat table template for you to print out and fill in.

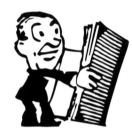

Smart Alec says
'Did you include the PCT? PCTs place all sorts of information demands on practices and while they may not be top of your list, you will need to collect information for them too. Practice information is the foundation of a whole range of information used by primary care trusts, strategic authorities, the Department of Health and even the PM himself. As with all foundations, I'm afraid that you're bottom of the pile, but equally, if the foundation's not right, the rest of the edifice will come a-tumbling down.'

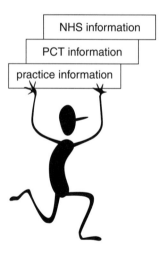

So, faced with the daunting responsibility not only of meeting the needs of your own practice, but of holding up the entire edifice of the NHS, what information should a practice system hold? The NHS prescribes standards for all systems to which all systems should conform, known as the *Rules for Accreditation* (RFA) for GP systems.

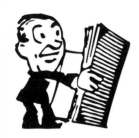 **Smart Alec says**
'The numbering of RFA is a classic of NHS common sense. First came RFA, then RFA2, RFA3 and RFA4. By then we were getting the hang of things, so next we got RFA99 in the year 1999, followed by what we thought was going to be RFA2001 in 2001. Instead we got RFA99 v.1.2. All clear now?'

This model has six categories of information:

- practice
- partners and staff
- related organisations
- patient registration
- clinical record
- drug database.

Table 1.1 shows the RFA99 v.1.2 information requirements in more detail.

Table 1.1   Information specified by RFA99 v.1.2 for GP systems

Practice information	The practice	• The name and identification number of the practice • The address(es) of practice premises including branch surgeries • Telephone (at least two) and fax/modem numbers (at least one of each) associated with the practice • E-mail addresses for the practice and individuals within it • The PCG/PCT code • PCT site code, if applicable
	Partners and staff	• Their name and a nationally recognised identification number • GMC code and GMP code for partners, including the check digit (where appropriate) (*see* CO.A.1) • GMC code for other doctors, including the check digit (where appropriate) (*see* CO.A.1) • UKCC number for nursing professionals • Details of their professional role • Details of their contractual relationship(s) (employed by or associated) with the practice, including the start and finish dates of these relationships and an indication of whether or not they can prescribe
	Related organisations	• The name of the organisation • The code of the organisation (includes PCG, PCT, HA, Trading Partner, NHS Trust, private provider) • The address(es) of the organisation • Telephone and other contact numbers for the organisation • The e-mail address for the organisation • Names, departmental addresses and telephone/fax numbers and e-mail addresses for departments or persons within the organisation with whom the practice makes direct contact. These should be cross-referenced to Related Person
	Related people	• The name of the person • The role of the person (e.g. consultant) • The identification number where applicable (e.g. consultant code) • The address • The telephone number(s), fax and e-mail address • The organisation to whom they belong

Patient information	Patient registration	• Surname • Former surname • Forename • Title • Date of birth • Sex • Marital status • The NHS number (10 digit) • The old NHS number • Type(s) of registration • GMS – General Medical Services • PMS – Personal Medical Services • Child health surveillance • Contraception • Maternity • Temporary resident • Emergency treatment • Immediately necessary treatment • Private • Registration status • The registered home address of the patient • At least one previous or alternative address • Telephone or other contact numbers associated with the patient • Postcode • The responsible Trading Partner • The responsible Health Authority • GP registered with • The GP who usually sees the patient • The branch surgery normally attended • Carer • Date on which permission given for details of patient's carer to be entered • Whether the patient is a carer • Dispensing status • Rural practice information: mileage, walking units and blocked route markers • Date of removal
	Clinical record	• Medical, family and social history • Symptoms, signs and investigation results • Diagnoses, sensitivities and problems in terms of • A Read coded term, where available, identifying the characteristic

| Patient information (cont.) | Clinical record (cont.) | • A free text description qualifying or extending the meaning of the Read coded term
• The date on which, or dates between which, the characteristic applied
• The date of recording
• The system *shall* allow appropriate recall dates to be derived from other stored information such as age, sex, or the start of previous screening or treatment, and as specified by local or Department of Health initiatives
• The date on which the characteristic is to be reviewed
• One or more numeric values, where relevant to an observation or to the result of an investigation
• The person authorising the data entry
• The person recording (entering) the data (see CS.1.3.1)

All interventions carried out to investigate or treat the patient including: surgical, diagnostic and preventative procedures; direct access services, e.g. physiotherapy, occupational therapy, radiotherapy, psychotherapy, chemotherapy; counselling and health education; prescribing/medication in terms of

• A Read coded term, where available, identifying the intervention
• A free text description qualifying or extending the meaning of the Read coded term
• The person carrying out the intervention $
• An indication of whether the intervention was carried out by the practice
• The date of the intervention
• The date of recording
• The person authorising the data entry

Referrals and requests for investigation or treatment outside the practice in terms of

• The date of the referral or request
• The date on which requested action was taken
• The person making the request #
• The person or department to whom the request is made $
• The reason for the request
• The person authorising the data entry
• The person recording (entering) the data |

Prescribing and dispensing	Drug database	• Listed prescribable items including all products licensed under the Medicines Act (Prescription Only Medicines (POMs), Over the Counter (OTCs), General Sales List (GSLs)), all Advisory Committee on Borderline Substances (ACBS) approved substances and all items in Part IX and part X of the Drug Tariff
		• All such prescribable items listed product by product, with pack sizes, manufacturer, and an indication of the NHS reimbursement price
		• Cross reference to Read coded terms where appropriate
		• Serious and well documented/significant side-effects, cautions, contra-indications, interactions and active ingredient duplications
		• Doses, and indications
		• For items within the drug tariff
		  – NHS price (e.g. pack price, which would necessitate display of pack size)
		  – NHS prescribing status and legal category at pack and formulation level
		  – Black triangle status

Now that we've got an idea of the information that we need, we can start to think about designing a system to store and process it.

What's in a database?

The starting point for our design process is an entity-relationship model. Each entity in our model becomes a *table* in our database design. The next thing you need to think about are the *fields* you are going to use. Fields are the categories of information that your database is going to store. They correspond to the attributes of the entities that you define in an entity-relationship model.

Thus if 'patient' is an entity, then the attributes of patients that will become fields in our database include surname, forename, date of birth (DoB), gender etc.

Each patient in our system is an *instance* of the *entity* 'patient', and the data stored in the fields relating to a single patient make up a *record.*

Field types

Most database programs allow, or rather require, that you give each field in your database a *type.* The field type indicates what type of information is going to be stored in that field. Common field types are:

- integers (whole numbers)
- real numbers (decimal numbers)
- text
- dates
- boolean (or yes/no).

Microsoft Access also lets you store multimedia objects, such as pictures or sounds. Field types form a basic type of validation in that the database won't allow you to enter, say, text in a date field. They also facilitate sorting, as the database 'knows' more about the contents of the field. If you were to store numbers in a text field, for example, and then sort them, 11 would come before 2 because the character 1 comes before 2, and the numbers would be sorted in alphabetical order.

For a patient database, then, we would use text for the surname and forename, a date field for the date of birth and so on.

Keys

In order to produce a logical structure for your database, there should be something unique about each record in your database. This will normally be the contents of one particular field, called the key field. For example, in an ideal world, the key field used to identify patients in all parts of the NHS would be their unique NHS number, as no two patients should have the same one, and it should be recognisable anywhere within the NHS. This is in fact why the NHS is spending a fortune trying to ensure that everyone has just such a number.

Sometimes you can't identify a single key field in your database table. In cases such as this, you can create what is known as a *compound key* – a combination of fields that is unique. This can be any number of fields, but should be the minimum number required to produced a unique description of the record. In the patient database, for example, you could go for a combination of surname, forename and DoB. Even twins would be unlikely to have the same forename, but you might conceivably have two John Smiths with the same DoB.

Indexes

The final thing you can create for your fields is an index. Once you've started using your database, the data can be stored in the table in any order, probably the order in which you entered them. If you've got a lot of records in your database, then sorting and searching could take a long time. An index is just like the index in a book – it is an extra bit added on to the database to help the database program find records quickly. You are discouraged from indexing every field in your database as there is an overhead involved when creating the records, but you should index all key fields and any fields that you regularly use to search or sort.

Validation

Validation is the name given to the process whereby the information entered in the database is checked to ensure that it makes sense. For example, you can use validation to check that only numbers between 0 and 100 are entered in a percentage field, or only Male or Female is entered in a sex field. It cannot check that it is correct (the process of checking that the data is actually right is called *verification*).

Obviously it's very important that the information in your database is correct if you're going to get worthwhile results when you search or sort the data. There are various methods that you can use to check your data and these are shown in Table 1.2. You'd be amazed how many male hysterectomies there are out there in practice electronic records. Or maybe not . . .

What's special about a relational database?

So far we've only discussed having one table in a database. If we consider a simplistic database to record appointments, then we might consider three entities:

- patients
- appointments
- doctors.

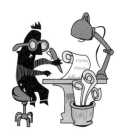

Over to you
Think what attributes you might need for each of the entities: patients, appointments and doctors. Record your answers in a table like the one below:

Patients	Appointments	Doctors

Table 1.2 Ways to check your data

Field types:	The use of field types forms a basic type of validation. If you make a particular field numeric (i.e. a number), for example, then it won't let you enter any letters or other non-numeric characters. Thus, a data listed as 34th March is clearly false and would be picked up as incorrect by simple validation. However, simply mistyping the 3rd of March as the 4th is more difficult to detect and must be picked up by a data *verification* process. Be careful when using the numeric types, however – if you use them for things like phone numbers, for example, you won't be able to enter spaces or any other sorts of formatting.
Presence:	This type of validation might go by different names, depending on your database program – sometimes it's called something like 'Allow Blank' or 'mandatory', for example. This type of validation forces the user to enter the data in that field. If you had an address book, for example, you might know the person's address and not their phone number, or vice versa, so it wouldn't make sense to make those fields mandatory. On the other hand, it doesn't make sense to have an address book entry with no name, so you should check for the presence of the name.
Uniqueness:	Some database programs allow you to check whether the contents of a particular field are unique. This might be useful to prevent users entering the same information twice. For example, if you were creating a car database, you should make the registration number field unique, as no two cars should have the same number.
Range:	If you're using a number field, then you might want to limit the range of inputs. For example, you might want to limit prices in a stock database so that they are all positive, or limit the range of a percentage field so that the values entered are between 0 and 100.
Format:	You might have a field in your database that requires an entry in a particular format. A simple example might be a date, or a piece of text of a certain length. More complex examples might include things like postcodes, or the NHS number. If you're using Access, you can define your own formats using an *input mask*, which defines the valid characters.
Multiple choice:	A good way to validate fields is to use multiple choice responses. These might take the form of a list box, combo box or radio button. For example, you could create a field that would only allow the user to select from Yes or No, or Male or Female. This can be an especially useful technique in database applications such as Access, which allow you to dynamically generate the choices. For example, if you created a database system to manage appointments, rather than checking the dates and times after they have been entered to check that there are no double-bookings, you could use a query and a combo box to show only the available times. That would stop you making double-bookings in the first place, and make any subsequent validation much simpler.
Referential integrity:	Finally, if you're using a relational database, then you can enforce referential integrity to validate inputs. This means you can check entries in certain fields against values in other tables. For example, in the merits database, when a new merit is entered, you could check the names of the students and teachers against the student and staff tables, to prevent either spelling errors or the entry of merits for students that don't exist.

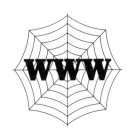

Web link
By now you should have gathered that you can download an Acrobat table template for you to print out and fill in, and are probably getting heartily sick of the reminders, so I'll stop!

You could put all of your entities into a single table, but think about what would happen as you enter the details for each appointment. For each new appointment you add, you need to enter all of the patient and doctor details each time. This would involve a lot of data being duplicated, and therefore take up a lot more disk space. This is known as *redundancy*.

As well as requiring more space and more time to enter, a number of other problems could arise. If you're having to enter all the details each time, there is a risk that you could make a mistake whilst entering some of the details, leading to, for example, a number of different spellings of a patient's name.

Using a relational structure allows you to enter the details of the patients and the doctors only once.

Searching (or queries)

Another advantage of a relational database is that it makes it much easier to query, or search, certain fields. For example, in our simplistic example it makes it much easier to query the database to find all the appointments of one doctor or patient.

Referential integrity

What would happen if you had two records in your database that were linked by a relationship, and then the foreign key or the primary key changed? Or one of the records was deleted from the database? The two records would no longer be linked properly, and 'referential integrity' would be lost (i.e. the rules governing how the data are related have been broken).

There are two ways around this problem. The simplest thing would be to stop the user making any change that would threaten referential integrity. You may have already noticed that Access won't let you delete information from a linked field, or enter information that would prevent it from being linked to another table (e.g. in our patient database, it won't let you enter appointments for patients or doctors who don't exist in the patient and doctor tables). However, some database programs allow you to 'cascade' any change to keys to other tables, so that if you change a key field, the matching fields in other tables are also changed.

Normalisation

The process of refining the structure of a database to minimise redundancy and improve integrity is called *normalisation*. When a database has been normalised, it is said to be in *normal form*. In theory, there are three normal forms.

Table 1.3   Normalisation and the three normal forms

First Normal Form	A database is in first normal form if there are no repeated fields. That means that there must only be one field for each item of data you want to include.
Second Normal Form	A database is said to be in second normal form if it: • is already in first normal form • has no fields that aren't dependent on the whole of the key.
Third Normal Form	A database is in third normal form if it: • is already in second normal form • it has no non-key dependencies. By *non-key dependencies*, we mean that there are no fields that are dependent on other fields that are not part of the key.

In reality, when you design your database and think about what your entities (or tables) are going to be – if you pick the right ones it'll normalise itself. So now let's see how to do that.

Designing a database using entity-relationship modelling

In simple terms, an entity is a thing. Therefore entity-relationships (E-R) are about modelling things and the relationships between them. In strict terms, E-R models describe both data structures and their interrelationships. E-R models are attractive because of their simplicity. They contain only two elements: entities and the relationships between them. Entities may be specific real objects such as people or machinery, or abstract concepts such as services. The relationships between them are classified into a number of types, according to the number of entities involved. It is the relationships which seem a little complex at first.

Let's start with a basic relationship that we can understand: parents and children in real families. Parents can have more than one child, but children can only have one natural mother and one natural father (genetic engineering aside). We represent this in E-R terms by saying that a mother has a one-to-many relationship with children, and this is represented by a simple diagram:

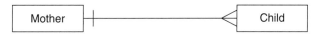

Figure 1.1 A mother-child relationship.

If we complicate matters a little and consider a woman-child relationship, then since the woman may not have any children (but a child must have a natural mother) this is now described as a one-to-zero-or-many relationship and depicted thus:

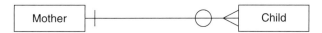

Figure 1.2 A woman-child relationship.

It is also possible to have a one-to-one relationship. For example:

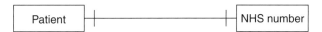

Figure 1.3 A one-to-one relationship.

The cynics may prefer the alternative view:

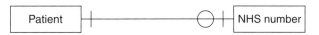

Figure 1.4 A one-to-one-or-zero relationship.

A further type of relationship is the many-to-many relationship:

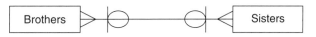

Figure 1.5 A many-to-many relationship.

A brother may have one, zero or many sisters and be the brother of one, zero or many sisters. Any form of many-to-many relationship is a bad idea for E-R modelling and should be broken down into two one-to-many relationships. We shall illustrate this process by use of an example.

For some reason, every course I have ever been associated with has taught E-R modelling using a video rental library as an example. In deference to the medical profession, we shall use the closely related example of a medical library.

At its simplest, a library brings together borrowers and titles. Each borrower may have zero, one or many titles on loan at any one time and although each copy may only be in one place at one time, each title may have more than one copy. Furthermore, if our model is to take account of time, we must allow that each copy may be on loan to many people. Thus we have a many-to-many relationship at the heart of our initial model:

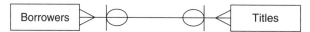

Figure 1.6 The many-to-many relationship at the heart of our library.

To break down this complex relationship we introduce a transaction entity. The transaction entity has the following properties:

- each transaction is unique
- borrowers may have many transactions, but each transaction may have only one borrower
- titles may have many transactions, but each transaction may have only one title.

Our model now looks like this:

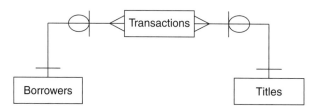

Figure 1.7 A simplified version of the library.

In practice, of course, life is more complicated than this. Each title may have more than one copy:

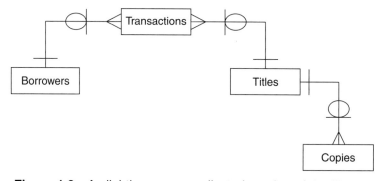

Figure 1.8 A slightly more complicated version of the library.

We can continue to take account of more entities, but we shall break off to consider the data which is required to describe each entity. These data are known as the fields, and each entity must have at least one which is uniquely able to identify each instance of that entity. This is known as the key. Note the following:

1 Every entity includes the key fields of those entities to which they are related.
2 The key for the copy number is an example of a multiple key. To uniquely identify a copy, you must use both the ISBN and the Copy number. Thus 'Copy 5 of Medical Statistics: a common sense approach' is uniquely identified by ISBN 0-471-93764-9 and the Copy no (5).
3 Unique identifiers may already exist: e.g. ISBN, NHS number, NI number. Where such standard identifiers exist they should be used: otherwise, an identifier may have to be assigned.

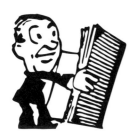

Smart Alec says
'Developers often suggest that E-R diagrams are simple and easy to understand.

• Do you agree?
• Do your colleagues agree?
• Do they understand even a simple unrealistic diagram like the one here? Could you explain it to them?'

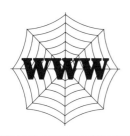

Web link
On the website in the Chapter 1 section you will find a multimedia entity-relationship modelling tutorial to download. You will need PowerPoint and sound on your computer to make much sense of it, but if you have these, try it and see if it helps you understand entity-relationship modelling.

In the next chapter we shall see how to turn our design into a real application.

2

Building a database

A very simple database

We're going to build a database. We're going to start with something very simple. The core business of primary health care remains the consultation between a clinician and a patient. Therefore we shall start with a simple application based upon an entity relationship of just three entities:

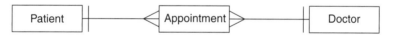

Figure 2.1 Simple model of a consultation.

To illustrate database construction, we shall use Microsoft Access^{TM}. This is because it is the application that you are most likely to have access to in the NHS (forgive the pun). First, we must construct a table for each entity. Then we must decide on the attributes of each entity to become the fields of the table.

Table 2.1 Attributes (fields) for our entities (tables)

Entity	Patient	Appointment	Doctor
Unique field (key)	NHS number	Appointment_id	GMC number
Other fields	Surname	NHS number	Surname
	Forename	GMC number	Forename
	Title	Date	Internal extension
	Phone number	Time	Mobile phone
	Address 1	Duration	
	Address 2		
	Postcode		
	Telephone number		
	Date of birth		

In Access we can create our tables from scratch or by using the wizards provided by the application. We shall use the wizards to create the basic tables, then tweak them to our requirements.

First, open Access by clicking on the icon: ⊠. The opening screen offers you a range of options. Select 'Access database wizards, pages, and projects'. Click on OK or press ↵ .

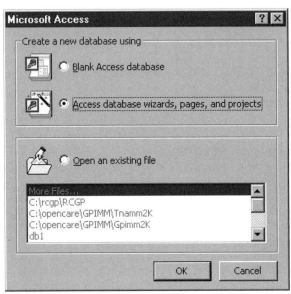

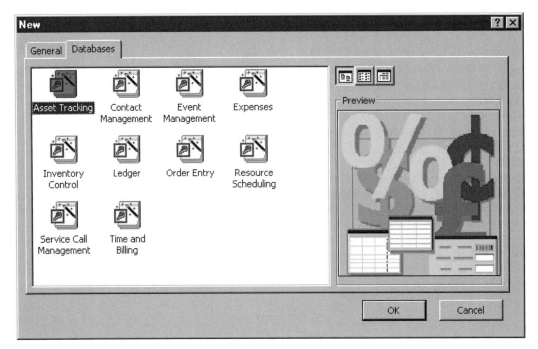

Click on the General tab:

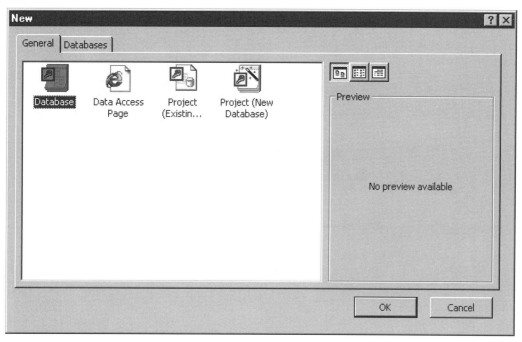

Click on Database and then on OK.

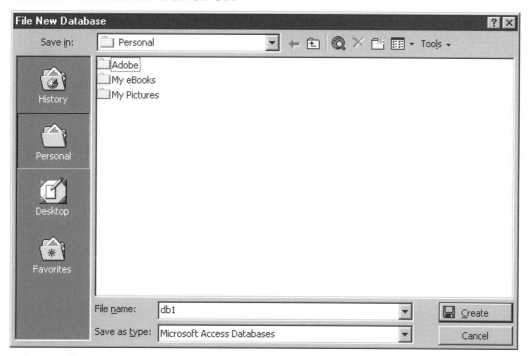

Click on Create.

Creating a table using the wizards

At the next screen select the 'Create table by using wizard' option by double-clicking on it:

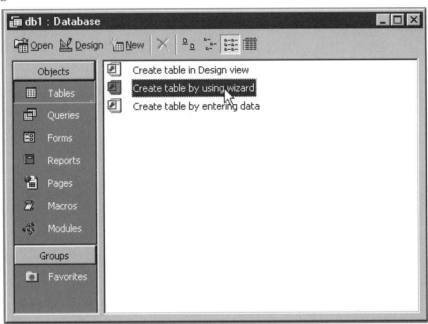

This brings up the first window of the wizard:

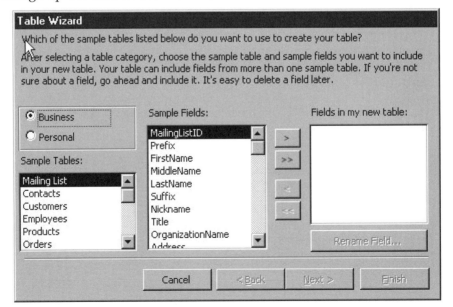

Select the business option.
    Select the Customers sample table.
    Select the CustomerID sample field.

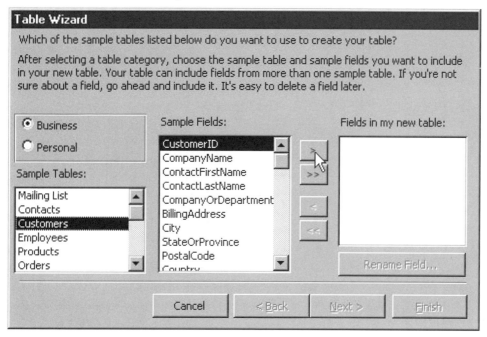

Click on > to place the field in the new table:

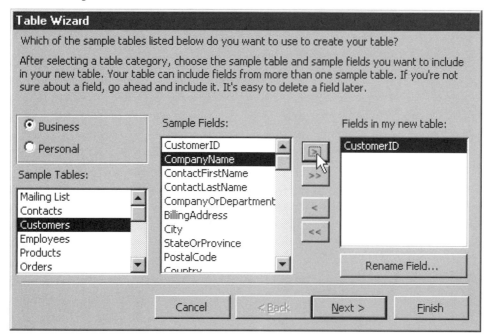

However, we deal with patients not customers in the NHS, so we need to rename this field. Click on Rename Field . . . and the Rename field dialog box appears:

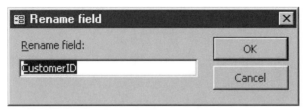

Type **NHSNumber** and it replaces the highlighted text:

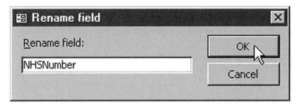

Click on OK and the new name appears in the main dialog box. Now repeat the process for the following fields:

Table 2.2 Fields for the patient table

Sample field	Rename to
ContactFirstName	Forenames
ContactLastName	Surname
City	Address1
StateOrProvince	Address2
PostalCode	PostalCode
Phone number	PhoneNumber

And the dialog box should look like the one (I prepared earlier) shown below:

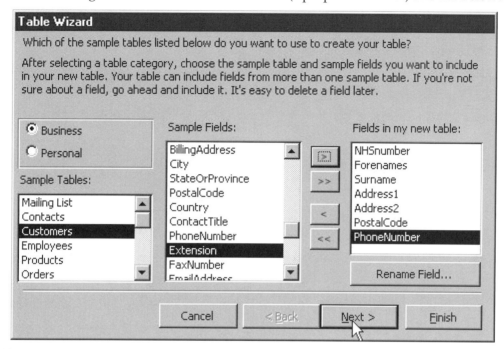

Click on <u>N</u>ext > and the system offers to set on your behalf or let you set up a key field and name the table.

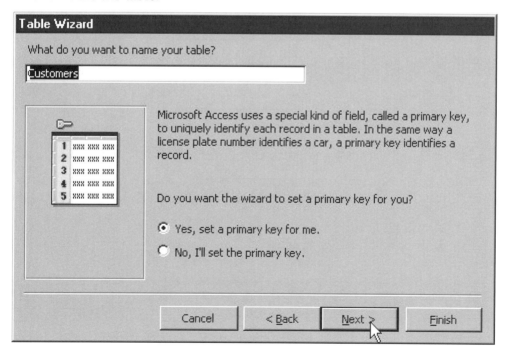

Select the 'Yes . . .' option and overtype **Patients** as the table name:

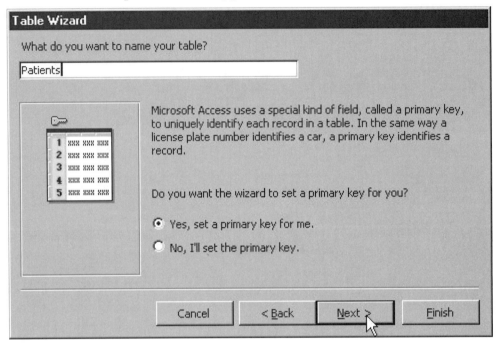

Then click on <u>N</u>ext >.

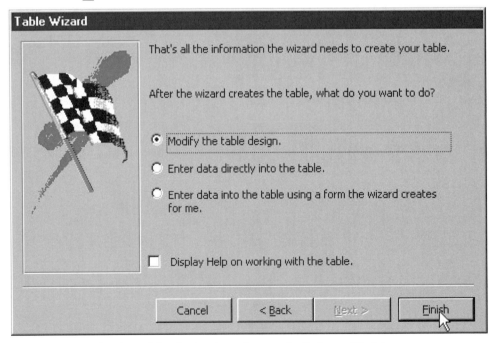

Select the 'Modify the table design' option and click on <u>F</u>inish.

You have created your first table.

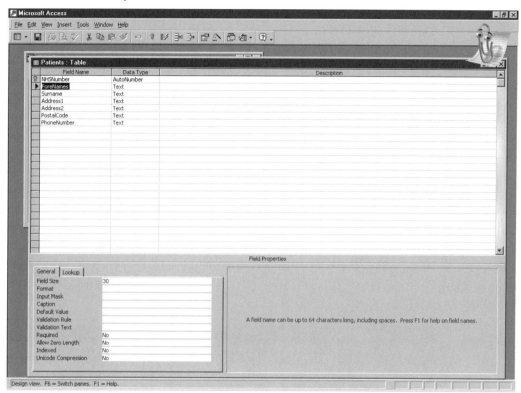

Now we need to add two more fields: Date of birth and Title.
  Select the first blank row if it's not already highlighted:

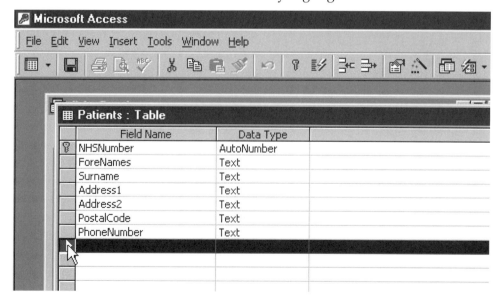

Click in the first column.
    Type **DateOfBirth**.
Click on the next column.

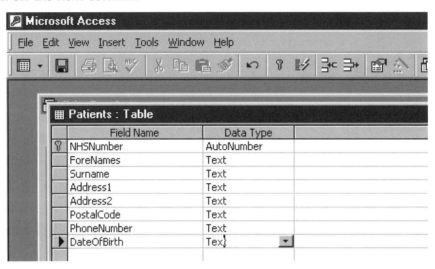

Select Date/Time from the drop-down menu that appears:

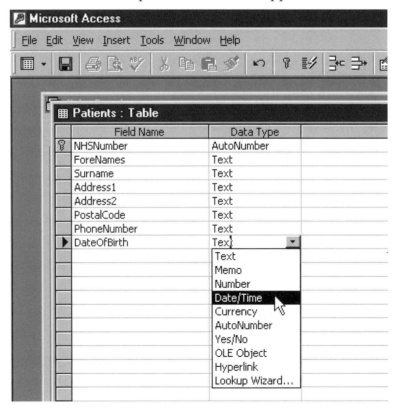

And the field type is set to date/time:

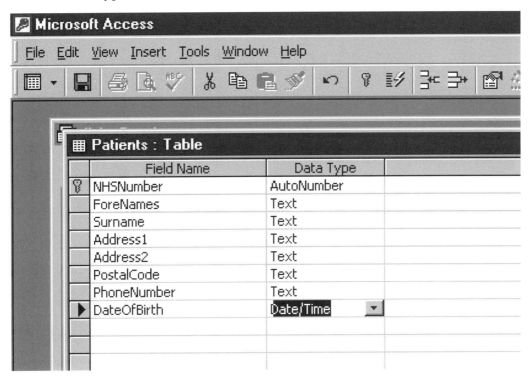

To control the way the field is displayed, go down to the layout box at the bottom and click in the format entry:

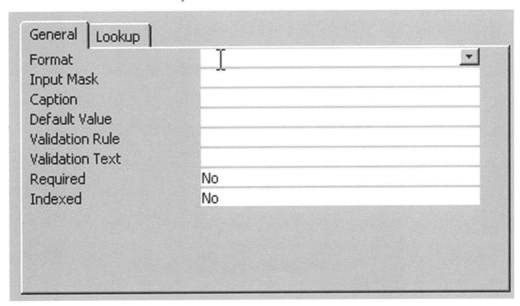

From the resulting drop-down menu, select Long Date:

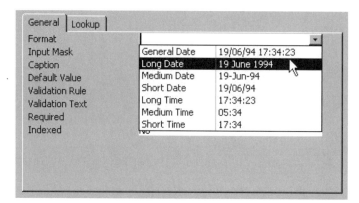

And this format appears in the main display layout box:

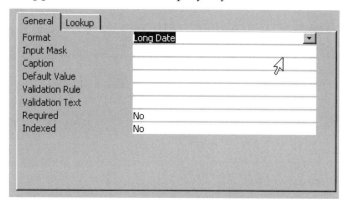

Now go back and add a title field as a text field type, using the first part of this procedure:

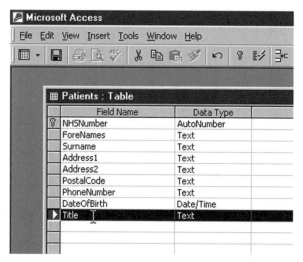

Our table is now complete. Close it by clicking on the **X** in the top right hand corner of the window. The system will prompt you to save your work:

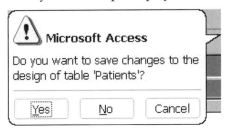

DO NOT FORGET TO SAVE YOUR CHANGES! You will be returned to the main database window and Patients is now shown as the first table.

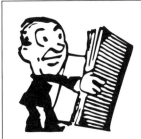

Smart Alec says
'If you click on the button in the top right hand corner of the application itself, the system will attempt to shut down the whole application. This can be very confusing, so please try and shut the table not the application.'

We will next create the Doctors table using the same wizard. I suggest you use the employees sample table and adapt it as follows:

Table 2.2 Fields for the doctor table

Sample field	*Rename to*
EmployeeID	GMCNumber
FirstName	Forenames
LastName	Surname
Extension	Extension
Workphone	Mobile

The new table fields should look like this:

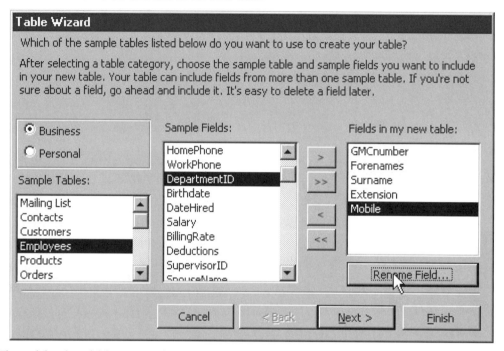

The table should be named 'Doctors' and the next dialog is one we have not seen before:

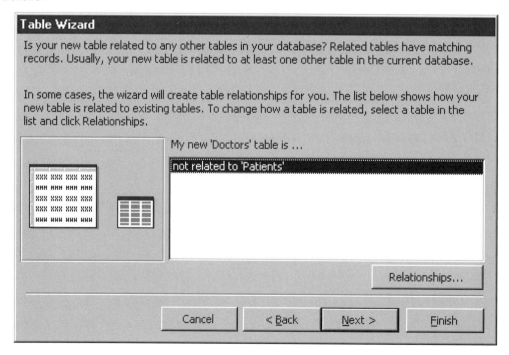

We know from our diagram that doctors and patients are not directly related so we accept this state of affairs and click on <u>N</u>ext > and then select the 'Modify . . .' option before clicking on <u>F</u>inish as before.

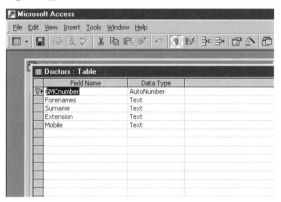

Once in design view, check it looks like the one above and then it can be closed without further modification.

Now we need to build our joining table, the Appointments table, and then complete the database by defining the relationships between the tables.

Building a table from scratch

The wizards are irritatingly American and oriented towards business rather than healthcare. Sometimes it's easier to do it yourself from scratch. We shall illustrate this for our third table, implementing the Appointments entity.

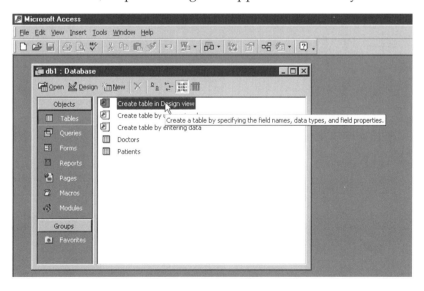

Double-click on the 'Create table in Design view' option. A blank table appears on the screen:

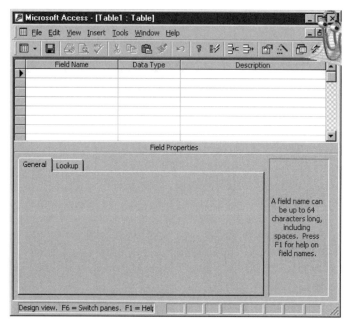

In the first row we shall enter our unique identifier, the key field. We shall use a field called AppointmentID and ask the computer to generate it.

Click on the first row of the Field Name column and type **AppointmentID**:

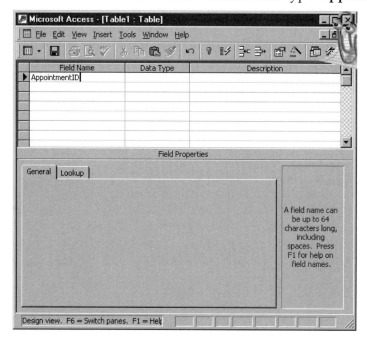

Now press the tab key to move to the Data Type column. We are going to use a field type of AutoNumber. This is defined as a long integer (a big whole number!) that automatically increments (gets bigger by one!) every time we add a new record. To do this, first select AutoNumber from the drop-down list:

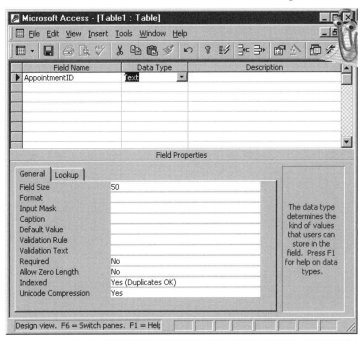

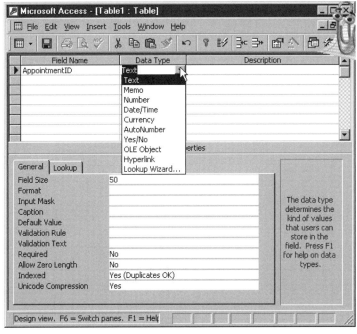

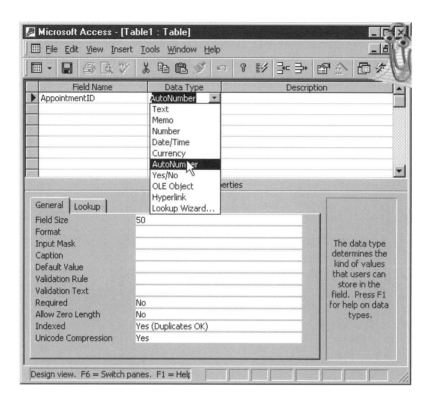

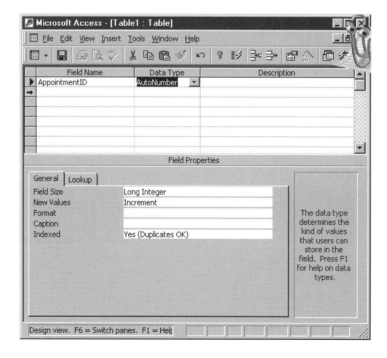

Now repeat the process for the second field. This is the patient identifier, for which we use the NHS number.

Click on the second row of the Field Name type and type **NHSNumber**. Then press the tab key to enter the field type. The NHSNumber is a string of numbers, so we accept the data type of Text without further ado.

Now click on the third row of the Field Name type and type **GMCNumber**. Once again, press the tab key to enter the field type. The GMCNumber is a string of numbers, so we again accept the data type of Text without further ado.

The next field is Time. Type the field name in the next row of the Field Name column and then press tab to move to the Data Type column. Click on the button to activate the drop-down menu, and select Short Time:

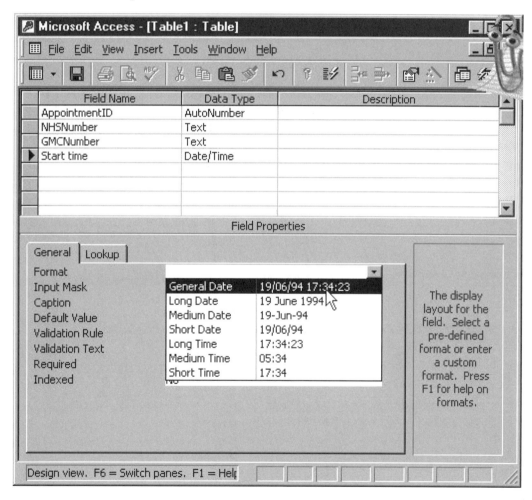

The final field is Duration. This is a numerical value, so enter the field name, then select number as the data type from the drop-down menu. When you have filled out this field, the finished table should look as follows:

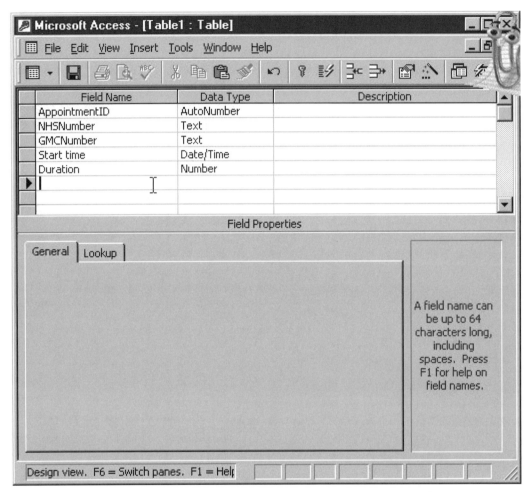

When you have finished, click on the Save icon to save your work.

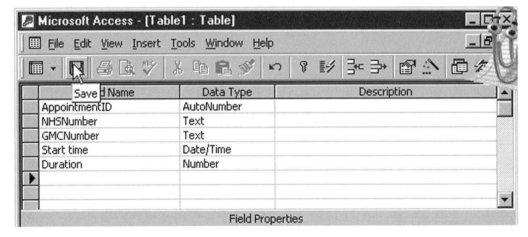

Now this table is finished and we have three tables. The next step is to join them up.

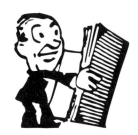

Smart Alec
Smart Alec has spotted a problem. Have you spotted it?
    If you want to spot it before we get to it, go back and look at the three tables. Otherwise, read on and all will be revealed . . .

Before we can join the three tables together we need to have fields that are identical to join together. Within the Appointments table, the patient is identified by their NHSNumber, which is a text string. Similarly the doctor is identified by their GMCNumber, also of text type. In the tables themselves, Access has assumed that these fields will be generated automatically as a sequence of numbers: 1, 2, 3, etc. Therefore, before we join the tables, we need to tell Access that these primary keys will be entered as text strings. We can still ensure that they are unique by specifying this. To do this, close the Appointments table by clicking on the X at the top right hand corner of the table window. At this stage, you will be prompted for a table name and asked if you wish to define a primary key. Answer 'yes' to both questions and name the table 'Appointments'.

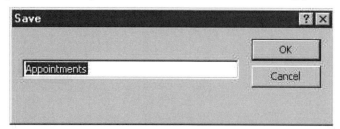

At the main window, select the Patients table and click on Design:

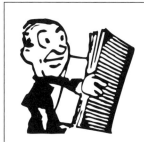

Smart Alec says
'If you double-click on the Patients table by mistake, then you will end up in data input view. This can be very confusing:'

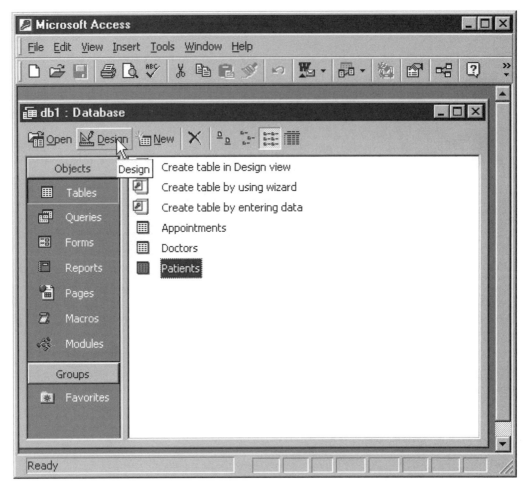

The table appears in Design view, allowing us to modify the field type of NHSNumber. Click in the field type of the top row:

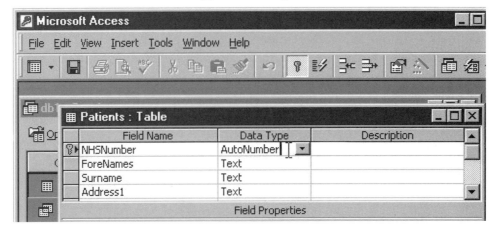

The drop-down menu appears:

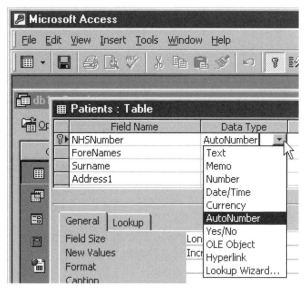

Select Text from the menu:

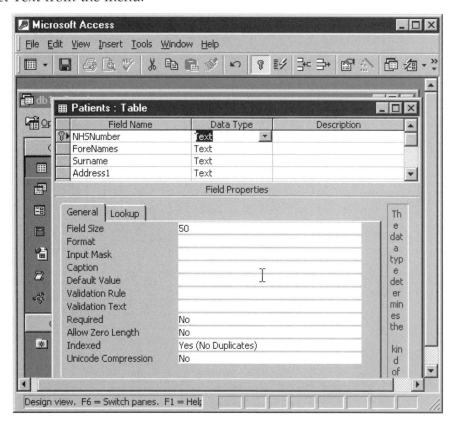

Now we need to specify a few field properties. Because this field was specified as a key, it is already indexed and this ensures that each value is unique. However, we must also specify that this field is required for all records:

Click on the Required property:

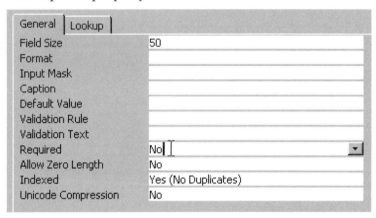

Click on the drop-down menu button:

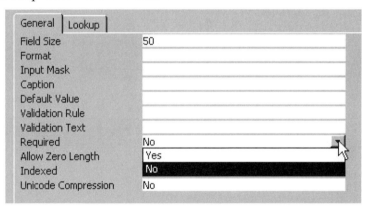

And then on Yes:

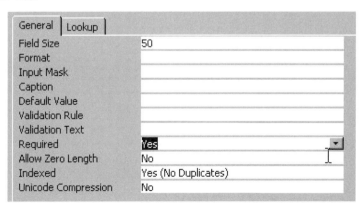

This is now complete. Click on the Save icon to save the changes, then close the window down.

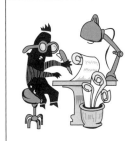

Over to you
The process of adapting the GMCNumber field type is the same as the NHSNumber. So it's over to you. For the finished result look below.

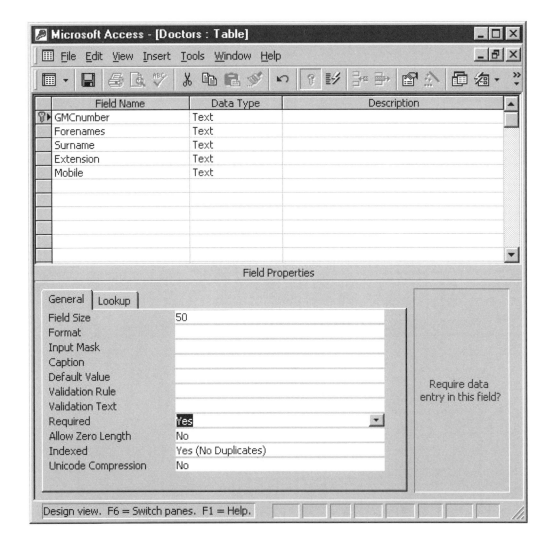

Joining up the tables

Now that we've got key fields that can be linked, we can define the relationships.
Go to the Tools menu and select the Relationships option.
The Show Table dialog box appears:

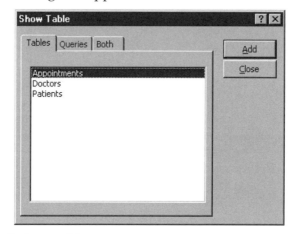

We need to add all three tables:

- Click on Appointments
- Click on Add
- Click on Doctors
- Click on Add
- Click on Patients
- Click on Add
- Click on Close.

The tables are represented in the relationships box:

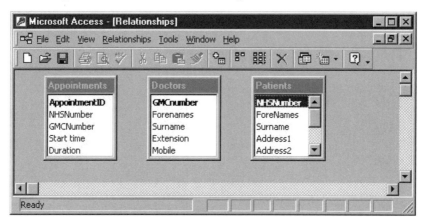

We can drag the tables around within this view: we need to put Appointments in the middle and Patients on the left. Re-arrange them so that they look like the screen below:

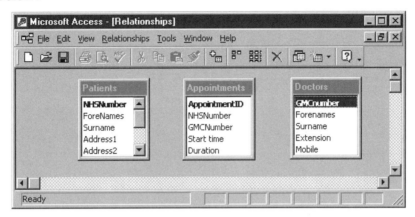

Now we can add the relationships.

Click on NHSNumber in the Patients box and drag it onto NHSNumber in the Appointments box:

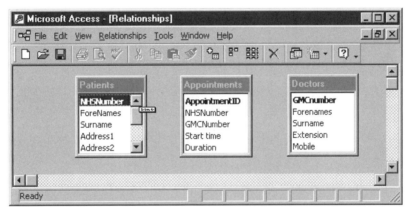

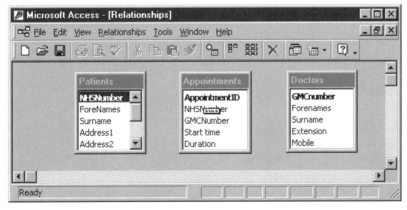

When you release the mouse, the Edit Relationships dialog box appears:

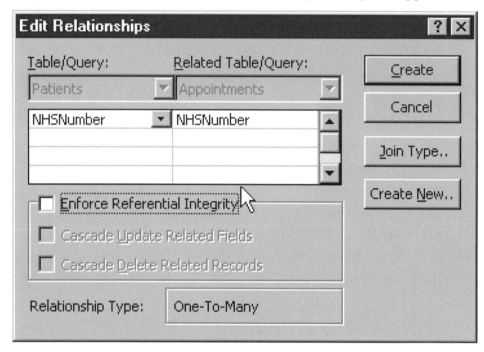

Check the 'Enforce Referential Integrity' box.

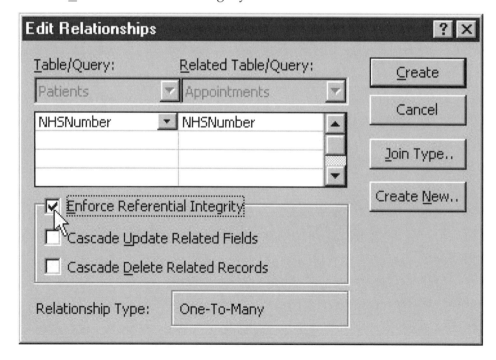

Click on Create, and the relationship appears in the main Relationships window:

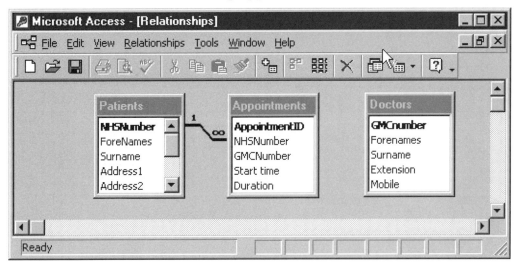

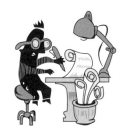

Over to you
The process of adding the link between the Doctors table and the Appointments table is the same as that of adding the link between Patients and Appointments, except that the link is made with the GMCNumber field instead of NHSNumber. The correct result is shown below.

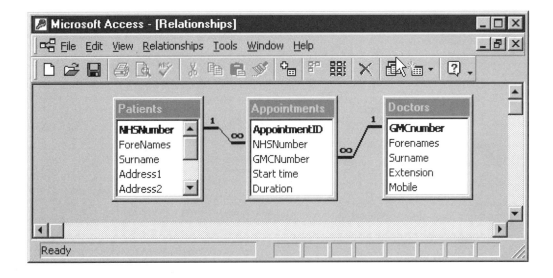

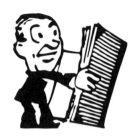

Smart Alec says

'Fancy that, you've worked through the whole chapter and ended up with something which looks jolly like where you started:

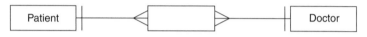

Spot the similarity?'

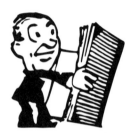

Smart Alec says

'If you want to test your skills, then try the following exercise:

Suppose the doctor wants to issue a prescription during the consultation. Modify the database to take account of this, adding an additional entity called Prescription and modifying the consultation entity accordingly.'

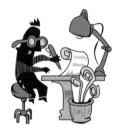

Over to you

1   First produce your entity-relationship diagram.
2   Then modify your database.
3   Save your new database as a separate application.

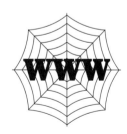

Web link

On the website in the Chapter 2 section you will find some model answers to Alec's little puzzle.

3

Populating a database

Forms

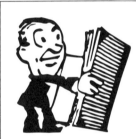

Smart Alec says
'You can put data straight into your database, but it's easier if you use a form. Forms provide a way of making data entry easier and also of adding extra validation checks. And if you're smart like me you can use them to build a whole application.'

Using the wizard to create a form

In the main database window, click on Forms.

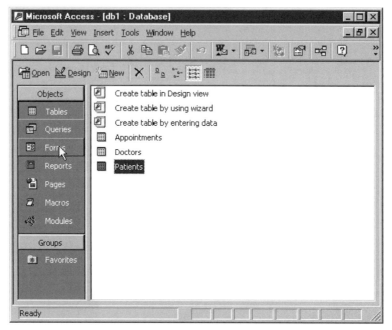

Then double-click on 'Create form using wizard'.

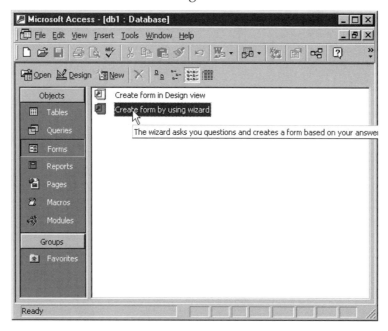

The first dialog box of the Form Wizard appears:

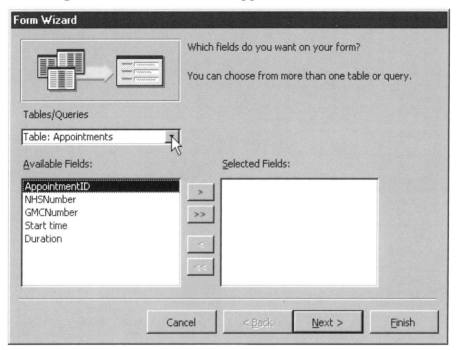

We shall start with the Patients form from the Patients table.
Click on the drop-down menu and then select the Patients table:

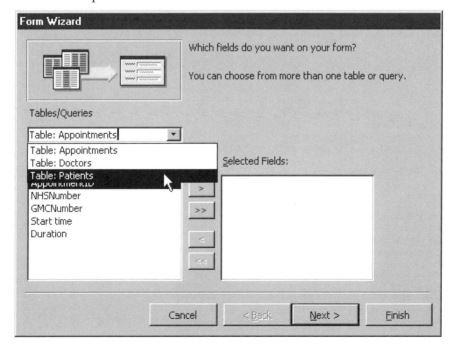

The fields from the Patients table appear on the left:

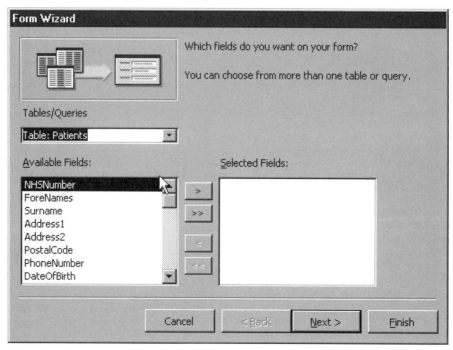

Click on ≫ to select all the fields.

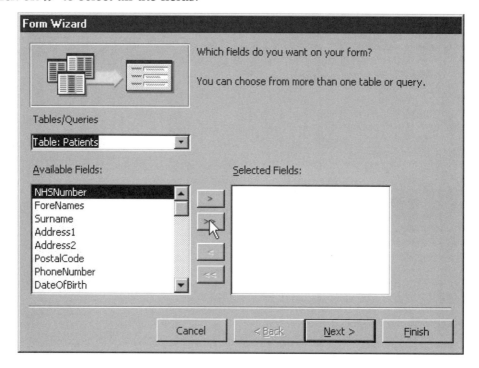

All the fields move into the right (Selected Fields) box:

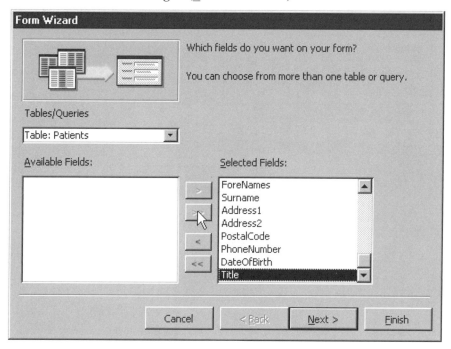

Click on Next >.

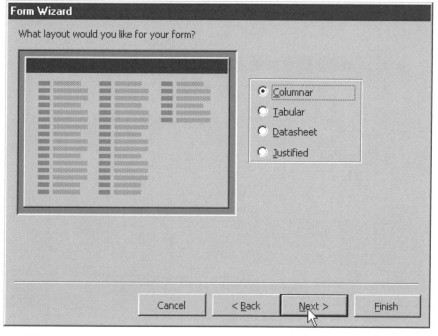

Select the Columnar option.

Click on Next >.

The next dialog allows you to choose from a range of 'looks'. Select a few different options, then click on Standard.

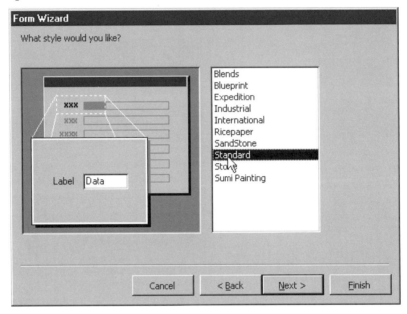

Click on Next >.

Almost there! This is the final dialog box.

Type in Patients as the form name and select the 'Modify the form's design' option.

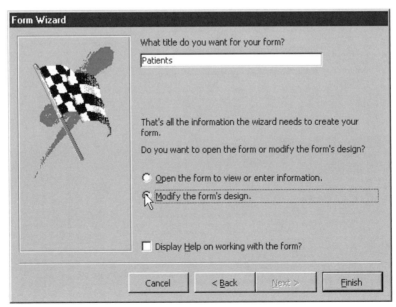

Click on Finish.

The form appears in design view. Each element of the form can be modified or deleted.

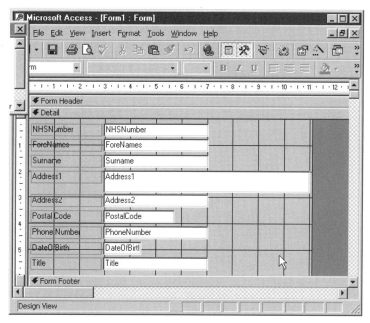

Let's try and make the form a little more friendly. Let's work on the title and names fields.

First, click on the ForeNames label.

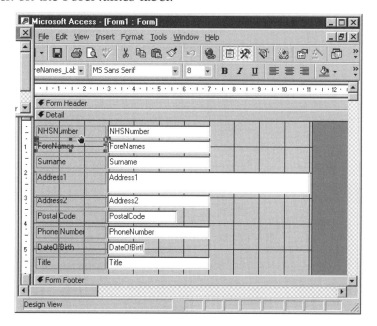

Next, click on ForeNames to edit the label and delete the word 'ForeNames' with the backspace key.

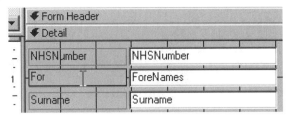

Now type the new label **Patient**. If you make a typing error you can correct it!

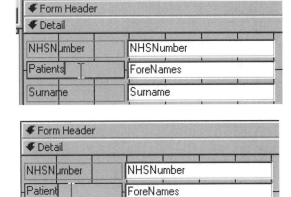

Next we're going to remove the Surname label.
   Select it.

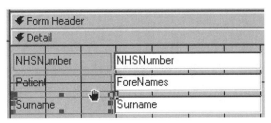

and then press the [Del] key! Gone!
   Next, select the data box Surname:

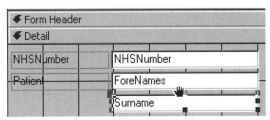

and drag it up and across next to the ForeNames box:

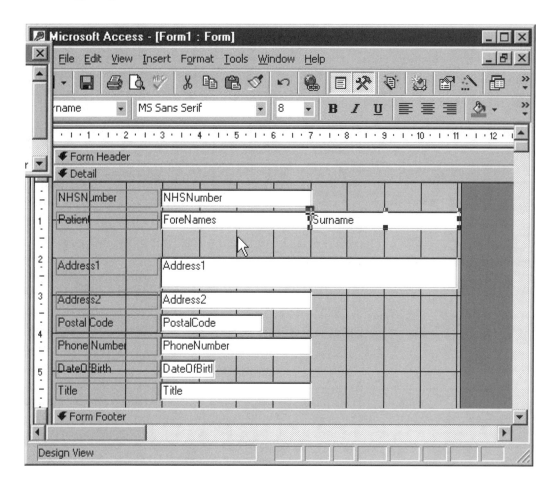

Logically, the title field should be up there too.

First, delete the label as we did for Surname.

Select it and then press the [Del] key! Such power!

Next, we must make space where it's going.

Click on the Patient label and drag the right hand edge to the left:

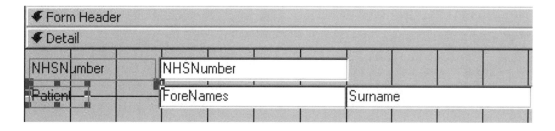

Now we can select our title data box:

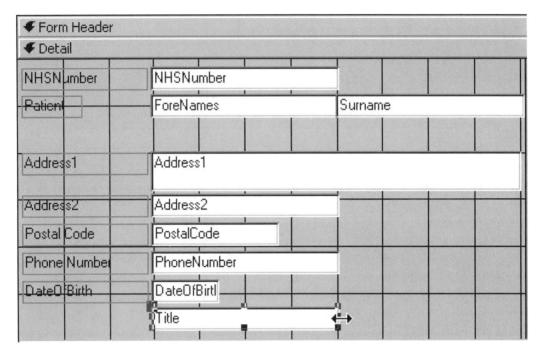

re-size it:

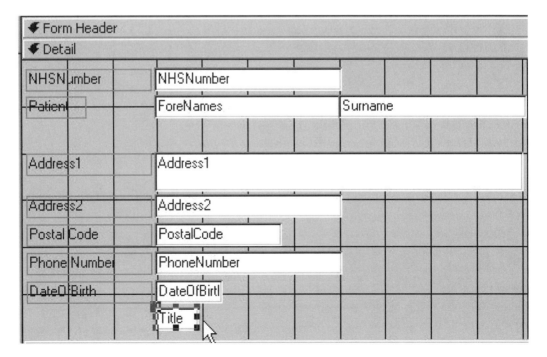

drag it:

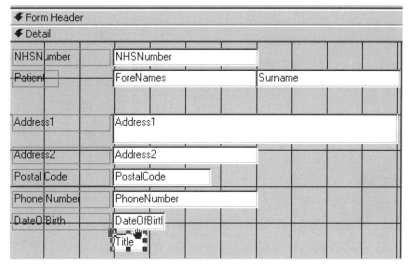

and drop it in the right place:

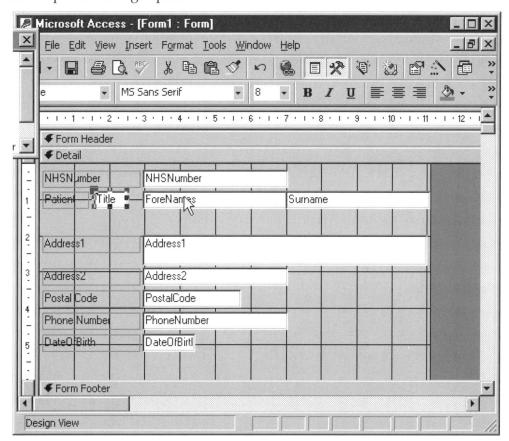

The last thing we'll do is move the fields down to make room for a title.

Select the top two rows of the table by dragging the mouse over them:

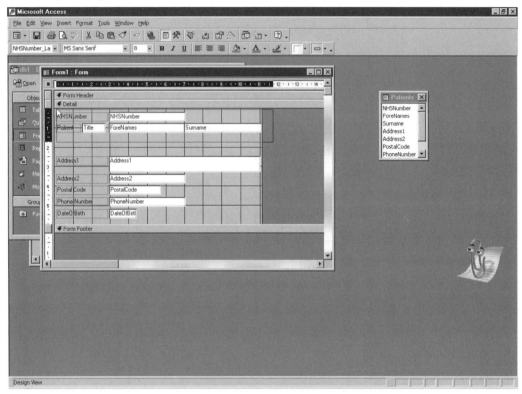

When you release the mouse all the elements are selected:

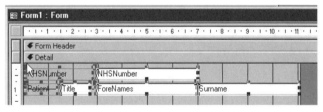

Now drag them down to close the gap between the Patient and Address rows:

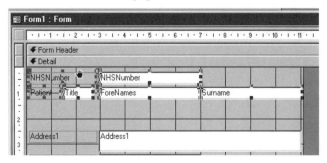

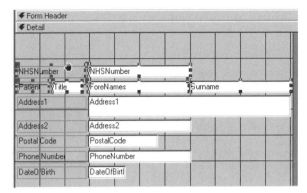

If we want to add a title, we need the toolbox:

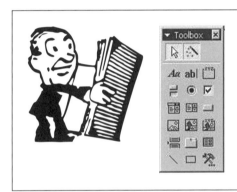

Smart Alec says

'This is the form tool box. If you can't find it on your screen look for the toolbox icon on your toolbar and click on it. It's the one with the hammer and spanner on it.'

'Psst, haven't you missed me? He's not let me in this chapter since the beginning.'

Click on *Aa* to add a label:

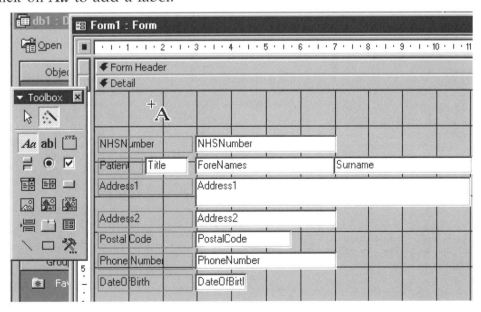

Drag a box where you want your title (I suggest you line it up with the data boxes) and then release the mouse.

Type your title; in this case, **Patients**.

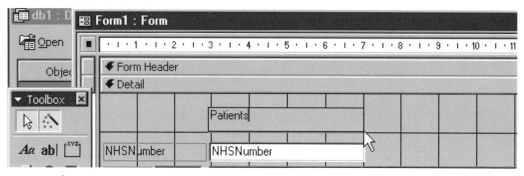

press ↵ when you have finished.

To change how the title looks, right-click on the title. The menu that appears allows you to change the properties of the title.

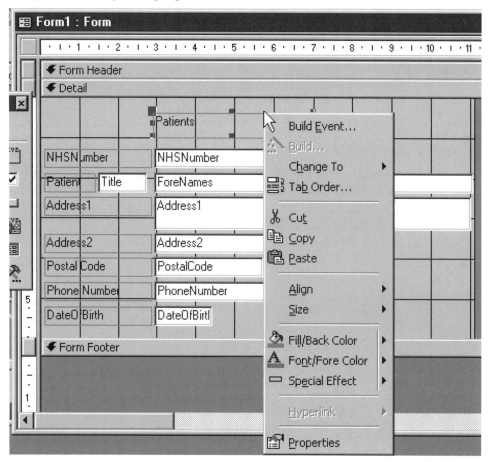

For example, to change the text colour to yellow:

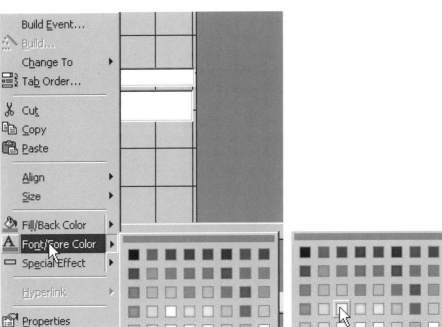

The last option on the menu is Properties. Here there be dragons: but dragons guard untold wealth! The Properties option provides access to a wide range of options.

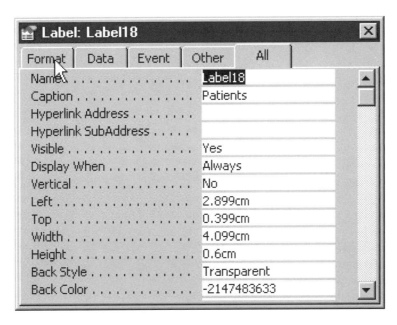

For example, to change the font and font size:

Click on Format.

Click on MS Sans Serif in the Font Name box (you may need to scroll down to find it).

Select Arial Black from the drop-down menu to replace it.

Click on 8 in the Font Size box.

Select 14 from the drop-down menu to replace it.

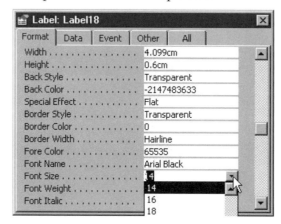

Close the menu and the results can be seen:

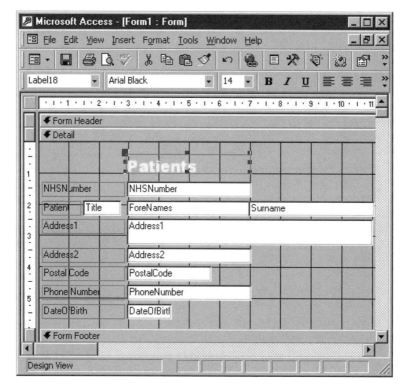

Now close the form and you will be returned to the main window. Patients is now listed as a form:

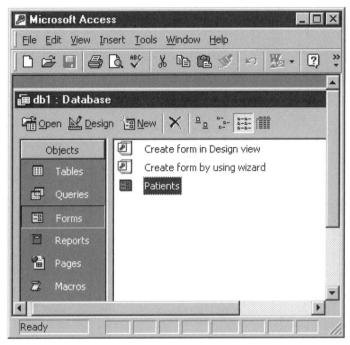

If you double-click on it you will see the results of your work:

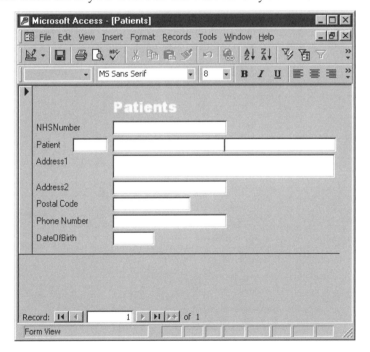

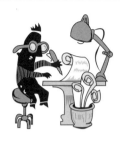

Over to you

Cue the theme music . . .

Your mission – should you choose to accept it – is to produce a similar form for the Doctors table. The process is very similar.

(This table will self-destruct in five seconds . . . only kidding!)

Here's what mine looks like in design view:

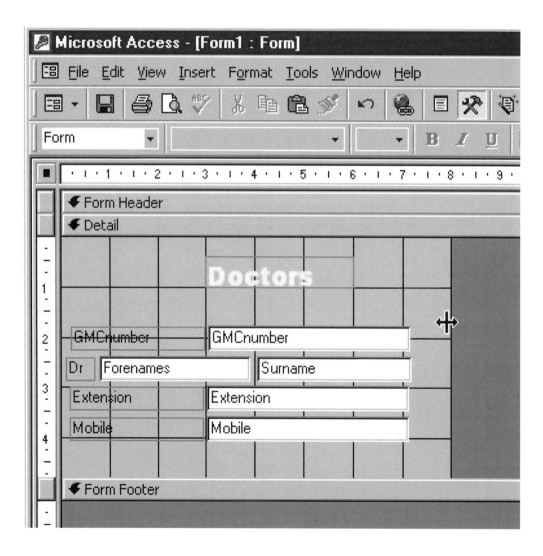

And here's what it looks like in data entry view:

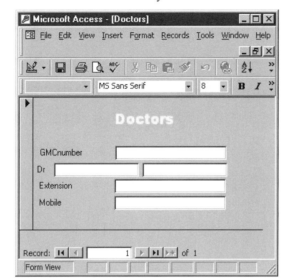

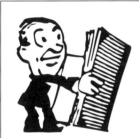

Smart Alec says
'Don't be afraid to play, and always remember: if you do something wrong, you can undo it either with [Ctrl]-z or by selecting Undo from the Edit menu.'

Designing an appointment form for data from more than one table

For the Appointments table, none of the wizards really meet our needs, so we'll design it from scratch. We shall also see how to draw in data from a number of tables into one form:

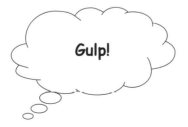

Gulp!

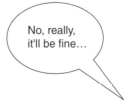

No, really, it'll be fine...

Start from the main database window and select the 'Create form in Design view' option:

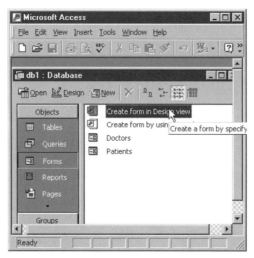

Start by adding a title. You've already done this for your previous two forms, so just do the same again, and you should end up with one like the one I prepared earlier:

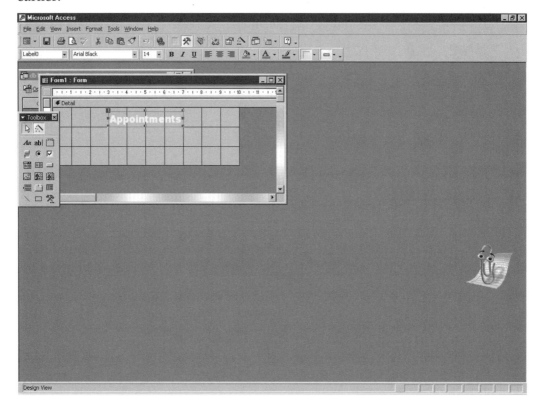

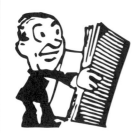

Smart Alec says
'Appointments is a big word. If you don't make the label box big enough, all your letters may not appear!'

Next, since the form itself looks a wee bit on the small side, drag the bottom right hand corner down and to the right:

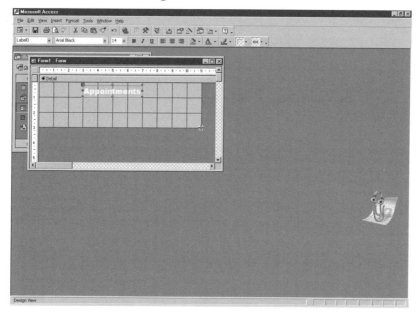

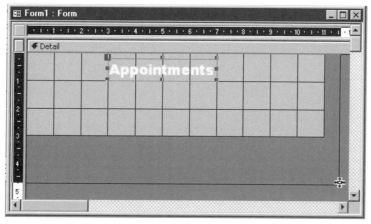

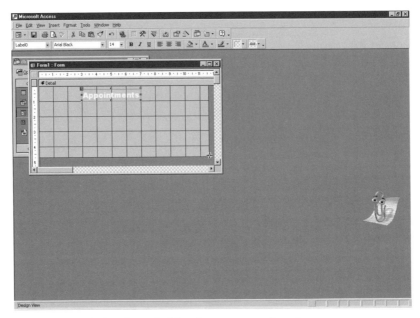

Now we want to add the four fields that we need to input:

- Date/time
- Duration
- Patient
- Doctor.

The first is a simple field linked to the Date/time field in the Appointments table, so we'll tell the form that it is based upon the Appointments table. Double-click on the form selector (that's the button in the top left hand corner).

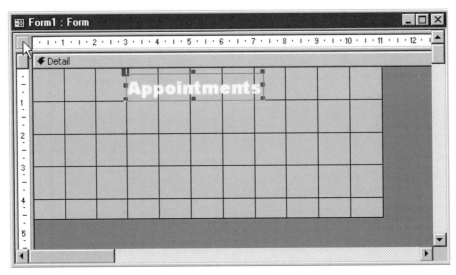

On the resulting dialog box, select the Data tab:

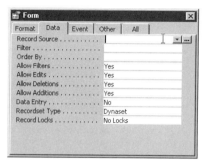

Click on the drop-down button and select Appointments from the list of available tables:

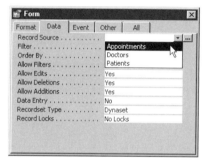

Now the list of available fields is available to allow you to tell the form which field you want to add. Select Start time from the list and drag it into position on the form.

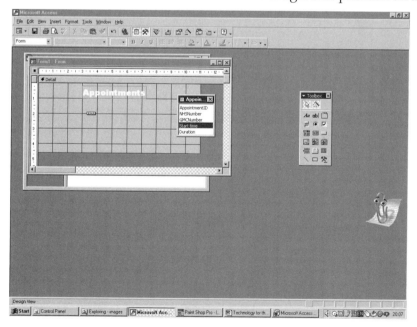

When you release the mouse, the finished box appears.

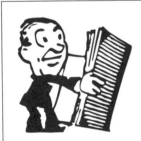

If it's not quite in the right place then just drag and drop it.

Smart Alec says
'This is known as a *bound* text box. This means that it is bound to a field in the table, in our case the Start time, and data entered into it will go into the table. If you try and put an unbound field in, the data has nowhere to go.'

The next field to be entered on the form is the Duration field. This field is used to record the planned length of the appointment, which may be 5, 10, 15 or, exceptionally, 20 minutes. We can use a combo box to select the appropriate values from a drop-down menu. Access kindly provides a wizard to help with this. Select Combo box from the toolbox:

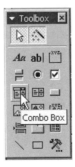

And then drag an area on the form where you want the box to appear:

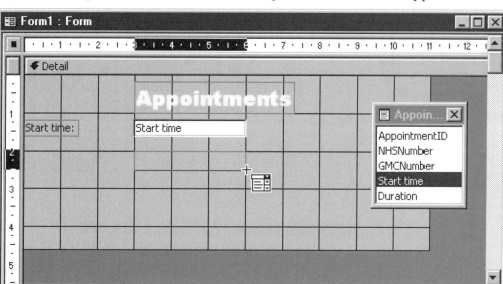

The first dialog of the wizard appears on the screen.
    Select the 'I will type in the values I want' option.
    Then click on Next >.

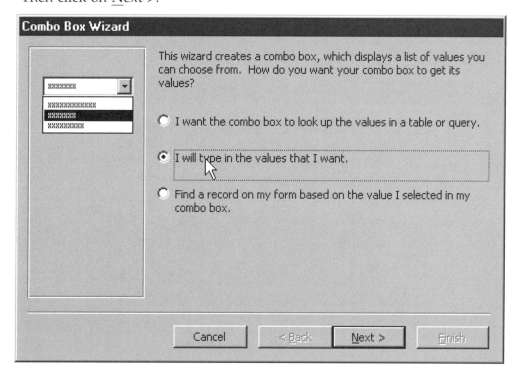

At the next dialog, enter the required values 5, 10, 15 and 20.

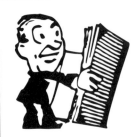

Smart Alec says
'Make sure you use the mouse or the Down Arrow key to move between rows. If you use the ↵ key, the wizard will assume that you have finished and move onto the next dialog. That's magic for you . . . haven't you ever seen Mickey Mouse in *Fantasia*?'

Before you move on, let's set the width of our drop-down menu.

Move on the right hand end of the column header, and then double-click:

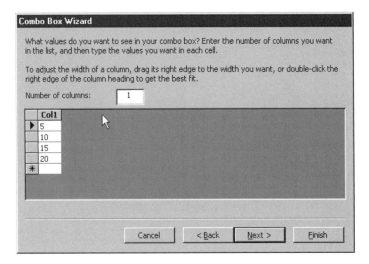

Then click on Next >.

The next dialog box allows us to select a field in which to store the data or, as Alec would say because he's a smart alec, bind the field. Select 'Store that value in this field' and then 'Duration' from the drop-down menu:

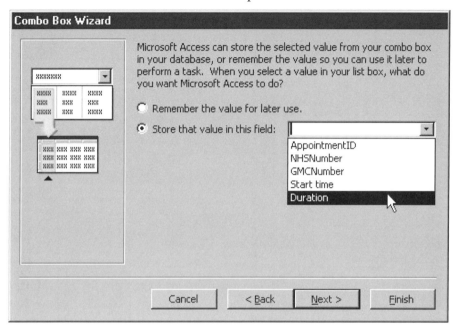

Then click on Next >.

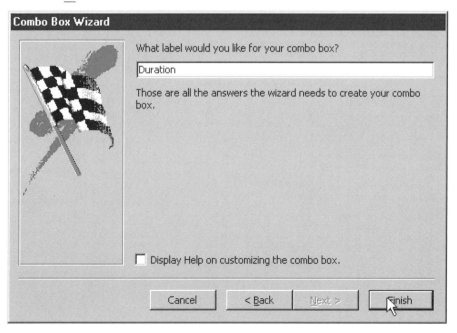

The final dialog selects the field name as the label for us, so we can just click on Finish.

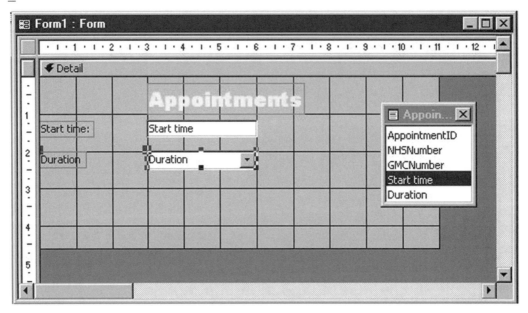

Now our form has two fields on it. Next we can add the patient. This starts in the same way, selecting a combo box from the toolbox and dragging it over to our form. However, at the next dialog, we choose the (default) 'I want the combo box to look up the values in a table or query' option by simply clicking on Next >.

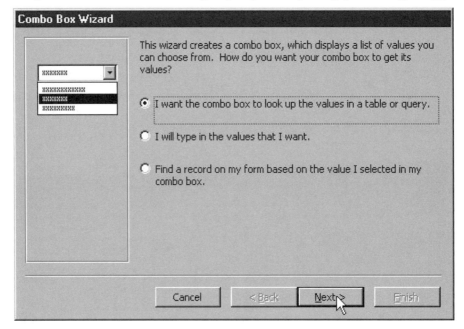

At the next dialog, we tell it to look up the values in the Patients table:

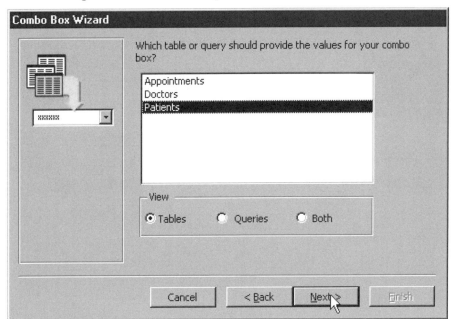

and then click on Next >.

Here we select the fields we want to use. First, click on NHSNumber and then select it by clicking on the > button.

Next, click on Surname and select it using the > button.

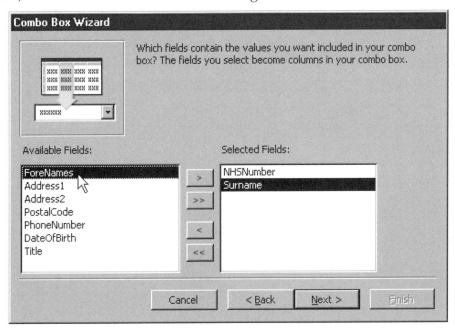

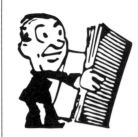

Smart Alec says
'Yes, he does mean *Surname* . . . he'll get back to Forenames in a minute and, no, it's not a mistake!'

Next, click on Forenames and select it using the > button:

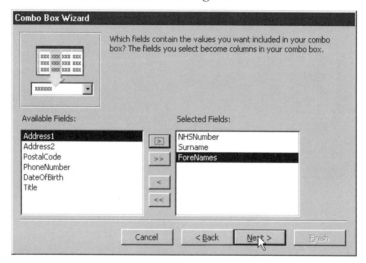

The next dialog shows us the menu with the surname first. This will be important later.

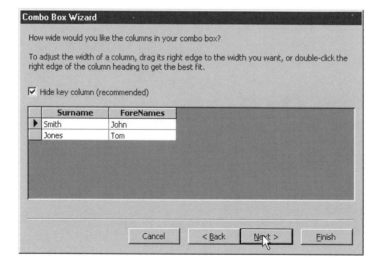

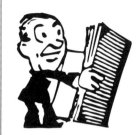

Smart Alec says

'He's cheated here because he's been into the table and added some data to show you how it would look. At this stage you've probably got blank fields.'

Click on Next >.

Now the steps are as before. Tell the dialog to store the value in the NHSNumber field by selecting 'NHSNumber' from the drop-down menu at the 'Store that value in this field' option:

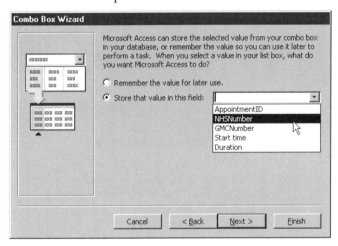

and then click on Next >.

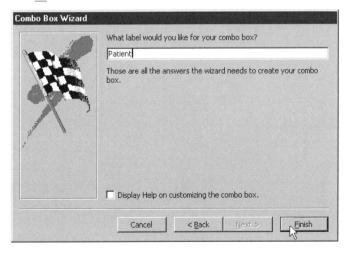

Click on Finish and the combo box appears on the form.

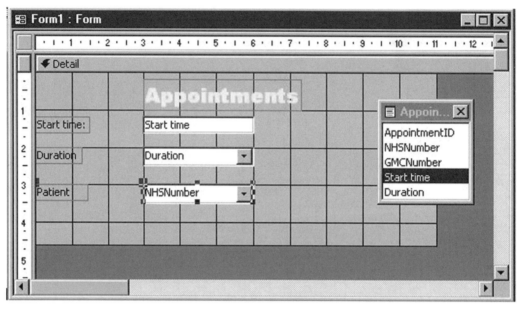

Now we need to add another combo box to put the doctor field onto the form.

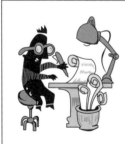

Over to you
The process is identical to what you've just done: link to two fields in the Doctors table, GMCNumber and Surname, and call it 'Dr'.

Hopefully, you will arrive at something like the form below:

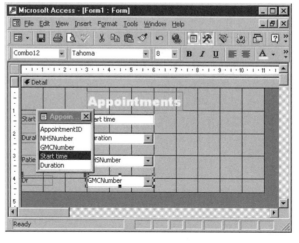

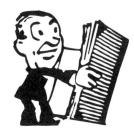

Smart Alec says

'Did you notice how we used the combo box to control the values that can be put into the Patient and Doctor field? The form will only allow you to set up an appointment for a patient and doctor already on the system.'

'Oh, and why did he do Surname first? Close the form, saving it as 'Appointments'. Next, put a couple of patients into the database and a couple of doctors. He used John Smith and Tom Jones for patients, and Drs Howard and Gillies. You will need to give them NHS and GMC numbers.'

'Now go to the Appointments form. In the duration box, you will be able to select from 5, 10, 15 and 20. In the patient box, you will see the patients you put in. When the box is shut, you see only the first field displayed. It seems more sensible for this to be the surname.'

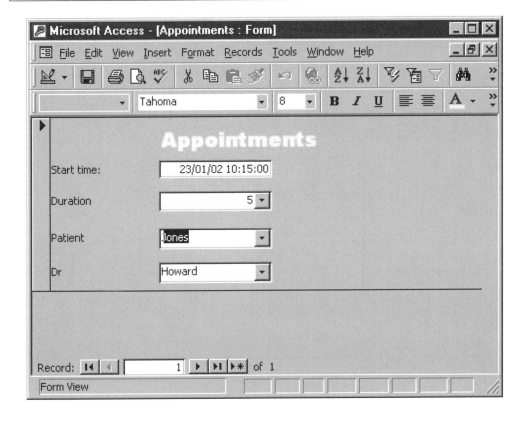

That's the form . . . probably it's time for a strong cup of tea!

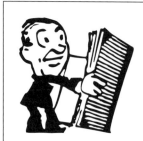

Smart Alec says
'The next bit is not essential. If you are uncomfortable, go onto page 88.'

Adding data validation rules

Using the combo box provides an elementary form of data validation. However, we can provide more. To see this in action, return to the Appointments form in design view. If you have it on the screen in data entry view, double-click on the view icon:

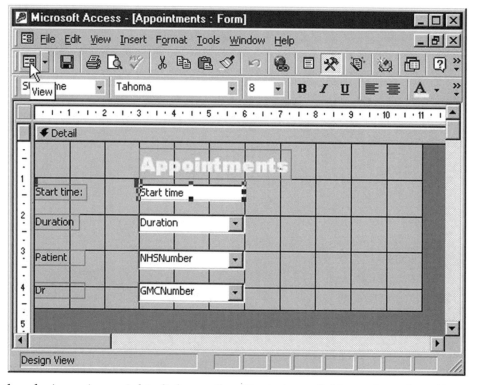

In the design view, right-click on the Start time field, and a short(!) menu appears.

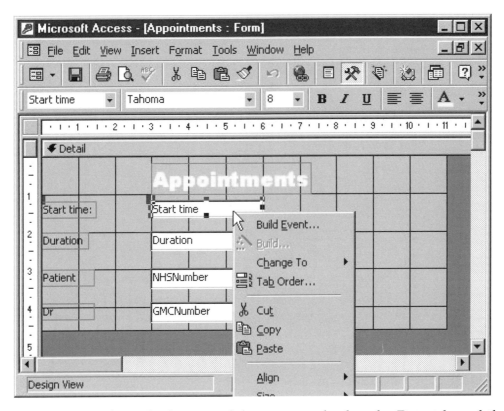

Select Properties from the bottom of the menu and select the Data tab, and the following dialog appears:

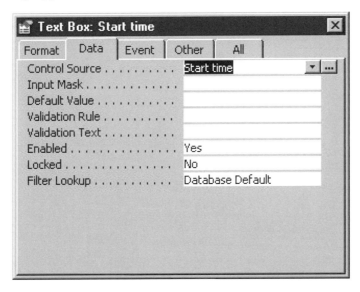

Click on the validation rule box and a button with three dots appears.

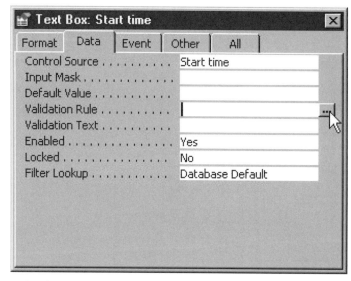

Click on this and a further dialog appears which might appear just a bit scary. We are going to tell the computer not to allow an appointment start time in the past. To do this, we have to use computer-speak rather than plain English.

'Do not enter an appointment start time in the past' becomes '> Now( )'; literally, 'Start time must be greater than the date/time corresponding to the current date and time'.

To do this, click on >.

Double-click on the plus next to Functions.

Click on Built-In Functions.

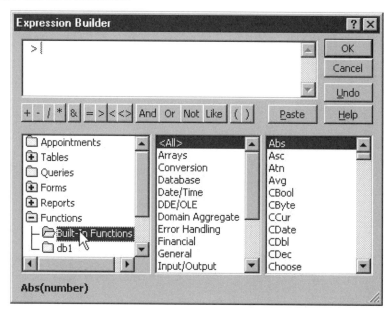

Next, we tell it to show us only the date/time functions:
Select Date/Time.
Scroll down and find 'Now' in the list of functions (the right hand list):

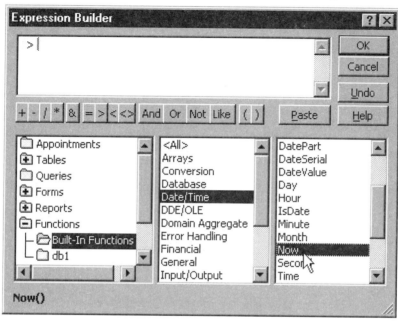

Click on Paste.
Now the expression is complete:

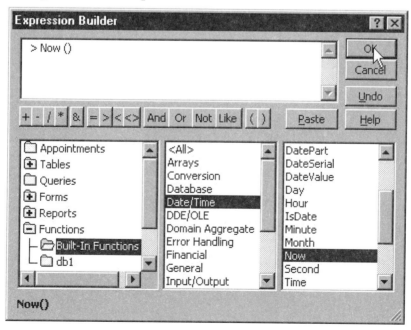

Click on OK to add the rule. Note that the rule appears in the validation rule box. Close the window to return to the form.

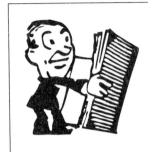

Smart Alec says
'To prove it works, click on the view icon again and try to input a value in the past in data entry view.
The computer should respond with an error message:

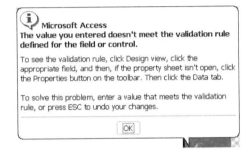

Using a form to build an application

We shall introduce one more form at this stage. It is a form to turn our database into an application by providing an opening screen.

First, create a blank form in design view with a title 'My first appointments system' as you did for the Appointments form. It should look like this:

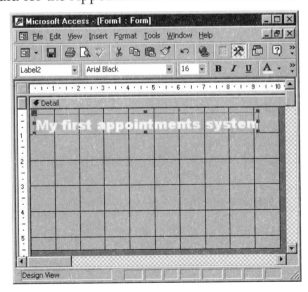

Next, we select the command button from the toolbox:

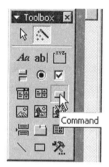

As before, drag and drop the button where you want it:

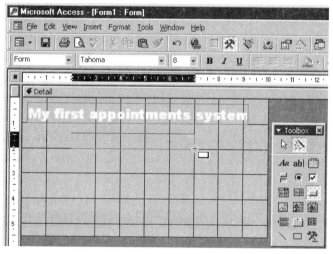

The first dialog of a wizard appears.
Select Form Operations from Categories.
Select Open Form from Actions.

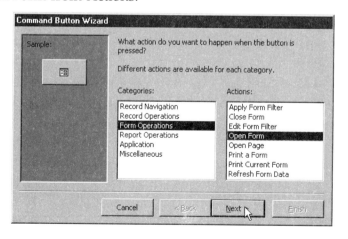

And then click on Next >.

At the next dialog, tell it to open the Patients form:

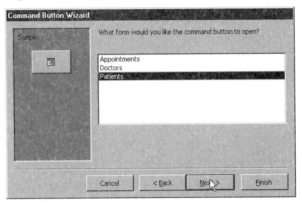

And then click on Next >.

At the next dialog box tell it to open the form and show all the records:

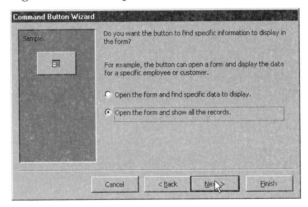

And then click on Next >.

At the next dialog, we can label the button.

Click on the Text option and type 'Add/Edit patients':

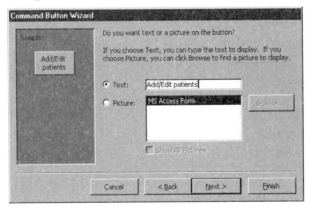

before clicking on <u>N</u>ext >.

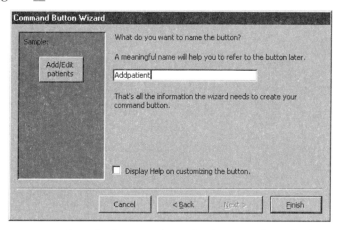

At this dialog, we can give the button by which it is identified on the form.

Type 'Addpatient' and click on <u>F</u>inish.

The finished button looks like this:

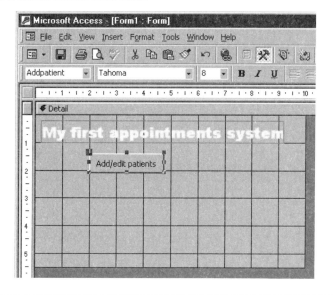

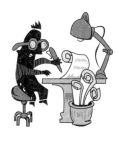

Over to you

We need to add two more buttons to add/edit doctors and to add/edit appointments. The process is identical to what you've just done.

Hopefully, you will arrive at something like the form below, although you may have to do a bit of re-sizing.

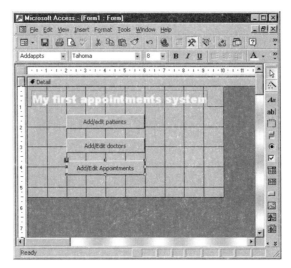

Next, we add an exit button. Again, the process is similar.

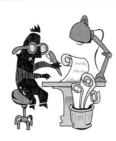

Over to you

Use the Command Button Wizard to create this button.

1 Use the Quit application command from the Application category.
2 Use the Stop sign picture as a label.
3 Call the button Quitapp.

Hopefully it will look like the one I prepared earlier.

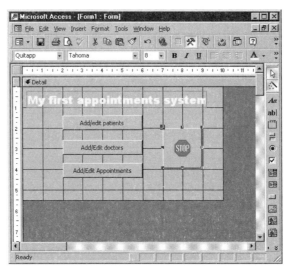

Save this form as 'openingscreen'.

Some finishing touches

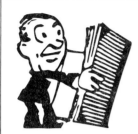

Smart Alec says
'One final point on forms. Sometimes the wizards can store up problems for you. Often these are caused by the American origins of the Access product. For example, read below about a problem with the Patients form.'

In the Patients form, we have recorded the patient's telephone number.
    Open the Patients form in design view:

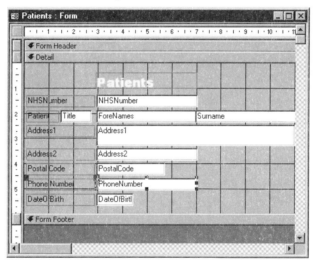

 Now right-click on the Phone Number box and select Properties from the bottom of the resulting menu. Click on the Data tab:

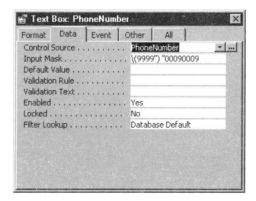

The input mask determines the correct format for the input string. The current mask matches a US phone number: a regional code up to 4 figures, then a 6 to 8 digit number. If you try to put in a UK number, you'll end up with a mess!

Click on the code and overtype with: \(99999")"0090009 'which expects a regional code of up to 5 digits followed by a number of 6 or 7 digits'.

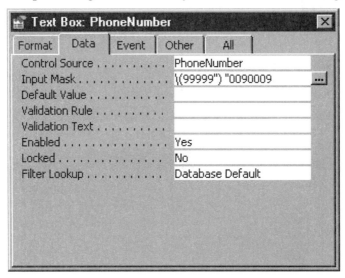

Now simply close this dialog to return to the form.

Now to finish off our application.

Go to the Tools menu.

Select the Startup option.

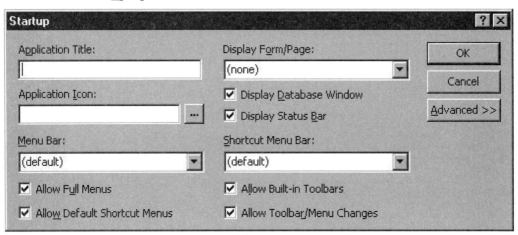

Enter 'My first appointments system' as the Application Title.

Select openingscreen as the Display Form/Page option.

Click on Display Database Window to hide this.

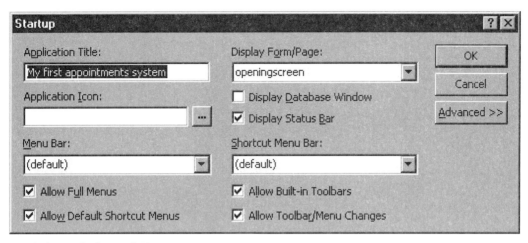

And then click on OK.

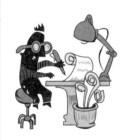

Over to you
Now make sure everything is saved, close the database and then return to it. You should find that the options you have selected are now in place and working.

4

Getting information out of a database

Queries

The whole point of putting stuff into a database is so that we can get it out again. Unfortunately, many people's experience is more of putting stuff in than of getting it out.

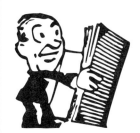

Smart Alec says
'Yawn, yawn, this is where he tells the elephant joke again. To save you having to buy another of his books or hear a talk, here it is:

"I say, I say, why is an NHS information system like an elephant?"

"I don't know, why is an NHS information system like an elephant?"

"Because we put lots of stuff into it, most of it disappears into the beast's gizzards, and what comes out the other end is generally a pile of dung."' '

In order to use our database, you will have to put some records in. I suggest that you put some patients, doctors and appointments into the system.

However, once you have played with it you may choose to use the populated database available from the website to work through this chapter. Alternatively, if you want to input the records yourself, the data are reproduced in the Appendix.

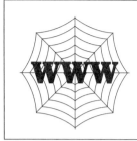

Web link
From the Chapter 4 section of the website accompanying this book you can download a populated version of this database.

At its simplest, the query allows you to select or sort a group of records.

Constructing a simple query using the wizard

To construct a simple query using the query wizard, go to the database window and select Queries.

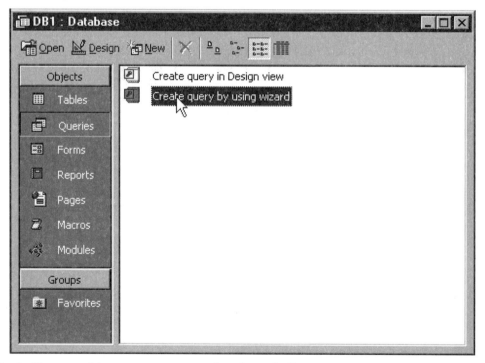

We shall start with a query to provide a list of all appointments sorted by doctor. Double-click on 'Create query by using Wizard'.

Select Appointments as the table to be queried. We are going to use four fields out of the five available.

Click on ≫ to select all the fields.

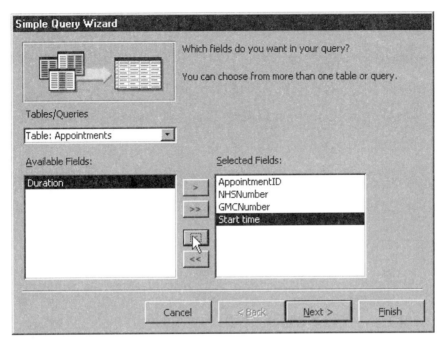

Select Duration and click on < to deselect it.

Click on Next >.

Accepting the title selected, choose 'Modify the query design'.

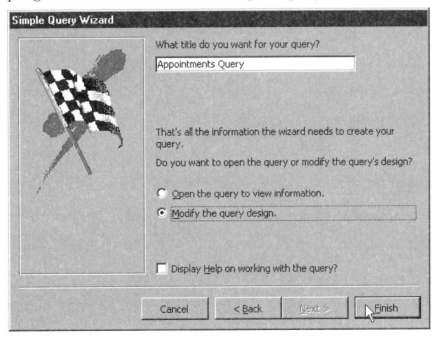

Click on Finish.

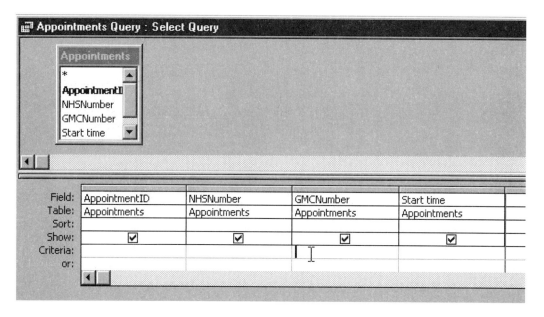

The design screen is in two halves. The top half shows the table to queried, the bottom the fields to be included. If we click on the Sort row in the GMCNumber column, then we can tell the query to sort the records by doctor in ascending order of their GMC number:

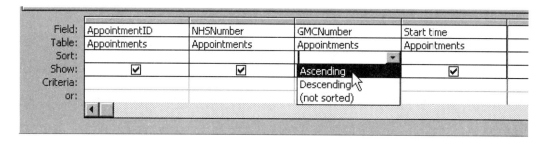

Click on the **!** button on the toolbar to run the query. The end result is utilitarian to say the least:

AppointmentII	NHSNumber	GMCNumber	Start time
1	450404	345789	/02/02 09:00:00
2	436771	345789	/02/02 09:05:00
3	203997	345789	/02/02 09:15:00
4	341884	345789	/02/02 09:25:00
5	556900	345789	/02/02 09:35:00
6	113679	345789	/02/02 09:45:00
7	202093	345789	/02/02 09:55:00
8	568797	345789	/02/02 10:05:00
9	104475	345789	/02/02 10:15:00
10	197099	345789	/02/02 10:25:00
11	644100	345789	/02/02 10:35:00
12	800340	345789	/02/02 10:50:00
13	471498	345789	/02/02 09:00:00

Record: 1 of 76

We can improve the results by using fields from more than one table. Close the query window. Double-click on 'Create query by using Wizard'.

This time select the following fields from all three tables:

- Start time from Appointments
- Duration from Appointments
- Surname from Doctors
- Forenames from Patients
- Surname from Patients.

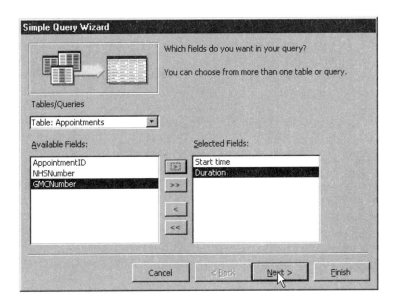

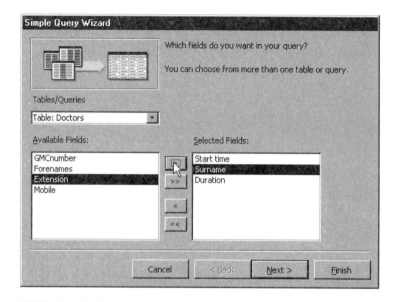

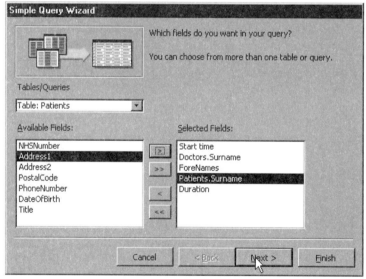

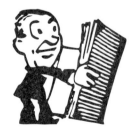

Smart Alec says

'Did you see that? Surname changed to Doctors.Surname when we added the Patients.Surname field to the query. I hate it when the computer starts getting smart.'

Click on Next >.

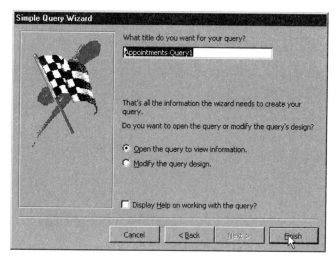

Accepting the name provided, this time we'll go straight to the query output by clicking on Finish.

The result is a lot easier to understand.

Start time	Doctors_Surna	ForeNames	Patients_Surn	Duration
23/02/02 09	Howard	Anna Mary	Croft	10
/02/02 09:15:00	Howard	Bruce Robert	Cross	10
/02/02 10:35:00	Howard	Tracy Emma	Elliot	15
/02/02 10:50:00	Howard	Ronald James	Evans	10
/02/02 09:00:00	Howard	Nigel Henry	Evans	10
/02/02 09:10:00	Howard	Elizabeth Cathe	Faulks	10
/02/02 09:20:00	Howard	Paul David	Francis	10
/02/02 09:25:00	Howard	David John	Davies	10
/02/02 09:35:00	Howard	Imogen	Davis	10
/02/02 09:45:00	Howard	Christine	Deighton	10
/02/02 09:55:00	Howard	Stephen Ivor	Dexter	10
/02/02 10:05:00	Howard	Mary Anne	Dobbs	10
/02/02 10:15:00	Howard	Lesley	Donaldson	10
/02/02 10:25:00	Howard	Sara-Jane	Edwards	10
/02/02 09:00:00	Howard	Robert Andrew	Crispin	5
/02/02 09:30:00	Howard	Harold Anthony	Franks	10
/02/02 09:40:00	Howard	Henry Cecil	Freeman	10
/02/02 09:50:00	Howard	John Paul	Gibbon	10
/02/02 10:00:00	Howard	Roger Brian	Gill	15
/02/02 10:15:00	Howard	Malcolm	Gillett	5
/02/02 10:20:00	Howard	Anna Elizabeth	Gillies	5
/02/02 10:25:00	Howard	Samuel Stephe	Goodacre	5
/02/02 09:00:00	Gillies	Anna Mary	Goodman	5
/02/02 09:05:00	Gillies	Simon John	Green	5
/02/02 09:10:00	Gillies	John Frederick	Greenaway	5
/02/02 09:15:00	Gillies	Catherine	Gurbutt	10
/02/02 09:25:00	Gillies	Graham Peter	Hailey	10
/02/02 09:35:00	Gillies	Arthur Stephen	Haywood	10
/02/02 09:45:00	Gillies	Darryl Wayne	Hill	10
/02/02 09:55:00	Gillies	David James	Hutchinson	10

Record: ◄ ◄ 1 ► ►I ►* of 76

Another way of using the wizard is to display basic descriptive statistics. For example, we can look at the duration of appointments by doctor.

Close the query window. Double-click on 'Create query by using wizard'.

Select Duration from the Appointments table:

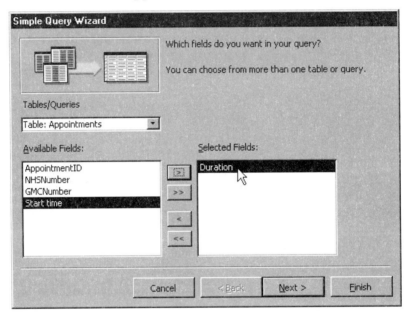

Select Surname from the Doctors table:

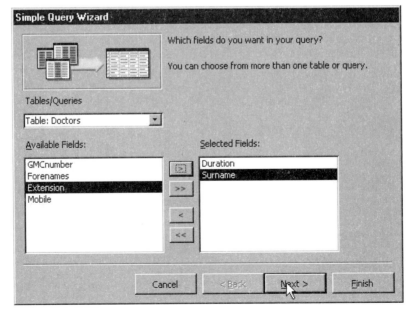

Click on Next >.

Select Summary.

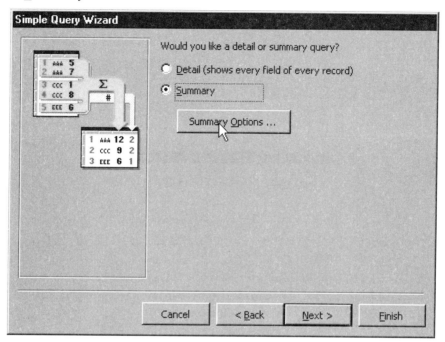

Click on Summary Options.
  Select 'Sum' and 'Avg'.
  Click on OK.

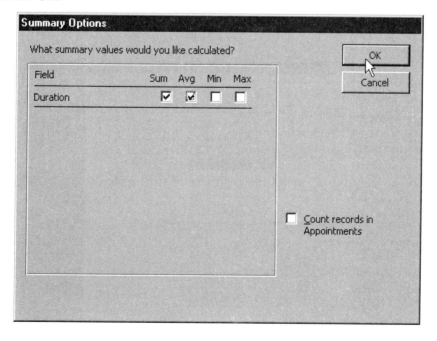

Accept the suggested name for the query and click on Finish to view the output.

Surname	Sum Of Duration	Avg Of Duration
Gillies	240	9.6
Howard	210	9.54545454545455
Shaw	260	8.96551724137931

The output shows that for the period under scrutiny, Dr Shaw had the most scheduled contact time with patients, but the shortest average scheduled appointment times.

Constructing a simple query in Design view

We can build much more flexible queries using the design view. Let's start with a simple query to pick out all the 15 minute consultations, sorted by doctor.

Close the query window. Double-click on 'Create query in Design view'.

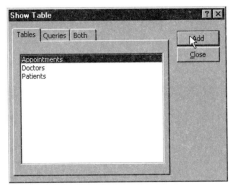

Click on Appointments. Click on Add.

Click on Doctors. Click on Add.

Click on Patients. Click on Add.

Click on Close. Notice how all three tables are now in the top half of the query window:

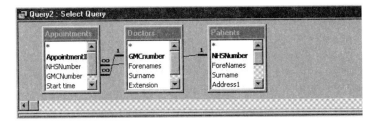

We are going to use four fields for our query:

- Surname from Patients
- Start time from Appointments
- Duration from Appointments, and
- Surname from Doctors.

In the field row of each column, select the field from the drop-down menu:

Field:	Surname	Start time	Duration	▼
Table:	Patients	Appointments	Appointments	Appointments.GMC ▲
Sort:				Appointments.Star
Show:	☑	☑	☑	Appointments.Dura
Criteria:				Doctors.*
or:				Doctors.GMCnumbe
	◄ ▢			Doctors.Forenames
				Doctors.Surname
				Doctors.Extension ▼

Next, we tell it sort the records by doctor in ascending alphabetical order of doctor's surname.

Click on the Sort row of Doctors.Surname and select Ascending from the drop-down menu:

Field:	Surname	Start time	Duration	Surname
Table:	Patients	Appointments	Appointments	Doctors
Sort:				▼
Show:	☑	☑	☐	Ascending
Criteria:				Descending
or:				(not sorted)
	◄ ▢			

Next, we tell the query to find all the records with a duration of 15 minutes.
Click on the Criteria row of Duration.
Type = **15**.

Field:	Surname	Start time	Duration	Surname
Table:	Patients	Appointments	Appointments	Doctors
Sort:				Ascending
Show:	☑	☑	☐	☑
Criteria:			=15	
or:				
	◄ ▢			

Click on the **!** button on the toolbar to run the query. The end result is shown overleaf:

Patients.Surname	Start time		Doctors.Surname
Patel	24/02/02	10:45:00	Gillies
Parkinson	24/02/02	10:30:00	Gillies
Parkes	24/02/02	10:15:00	Gillies
Lewis	23/02/02	10:45:00	Gillies
Gill	24/02/02	10:00:00	Howard
Elliot	23/02/02	10:35:00	Howard
Wilson	24/02/02	10:45:00	Shaw
Wilkinson	24/02/02	10:30:00	Shaw
Wilcock	24/02/02	10:15:00	Shaw
West	24/02/02	10:00:00	Shaw

Next we shall build a query to find all patients over 18.

First, select 'Create query in Design view'.

Next, click on Patients. Click on Add. This is the only table we need.

Select the following fields from the drop-down menus:

- ForeNames
- Surname
- DateOfBirth.

We have already seen the Now ( ) function in use in a validation check in a form. Here we shall use it in an expression to select only those over 18. Please note that this query was run on 5 February 2002. When you run it, the population will be older and you may get the odd extra patient.

In English, all patients over 18 are those for whom their date of birth is before the date 18 years before today.

In computer-speak, this becomes!

$$< Now(\ ) - (18 * 365)$$

This may be typed or assembled using the Expression Builder, which may be called into play by right-clicking on the cell concerned.

Field:	ForeNames	Surname	DateOfBirth	
Table:	Patients	Patients	Patients	
Sort:				
Show:	✔	✔	✔	
Criteria:			<Now()-(18*365)	
or:				

The result is as follows. No patients with dates of birth after 5 February 1984 are included in my results.

ForeNames	Surname	DateOfBirth
Tom	Jones	23 April 1954
Lesley	Donaldson	30 September 1917
Elaine	Smith	11 February 1961
Christine	Deighton	19 March 1940
Robert John	Peel	28 December 1952
Emma Jane	Abbott	07 June 1932
Colin John	Adams	29 May 1957
Stephen John	Aggett	26 June 1964
Naomi Catherine	Armfield	27 March 1950
Sara Ann	Armstrong	09 August 1973
Sally Christine	Atkinson	13 February 1952
Beverley Ann	Banks	25 April 1915
Jennifer Susan	Blaylock	02 August 1916
Emma Susan	Bowers	04 January 1932
Heather	Bowker	25 November 1974
Alan Graham	Briggs	17 February 1955
Kate Anne	Burrows	19 July 1914
Colin Stephen	Campbell	15 June 1968
Clive Stephen	Chambers	20 May 1916
Rachel Susan	Charlton	03 October 1921
Michael John	Christie	24 September 1919
Jennifer Cathryn	Clayton	24 May 1919
Christine	Clough	14 April 1983
Margaret Ann	Corbett	04 July 1956
Robert Andrew	Crispin	19 November 1957
Bruce Robert	Cross	06 November 1919
David John	Davies	17 January 1929
Imogen	Davis	18 June 1925
Paul David	Francis	12 April 1944
Stephen Ivor	Dexter	17 June 1975
Mary Anne	Dobbs	14 July 1923
Harold Anthony	Franks	05 February 1961
Sara-Jane	Edwards	26 June 1917
Tracy Emma	Elliot	04 September 1914
Ronald James	Evans	03 June 1942
Nigel Henry	Evans	14 November 1945
Elizabeth Catherine	Faulks	09 April 1972
Henry Cecil	Freeman	17 November 1936
John Paul	Gibbon	05 October 1948
Roger Brian	Gill	12 March 1927
Malcolm	Gillett	10 September 1922
Anna Elizabeth	Gillies	25 July 1951

ForeNames	Surname	DateOfBirth
Samuel Stephen	Goodacre	31 August 1928
Anna Mary	Goodman	02 July 1942
Simon John	Green	23 June 1928
John Frederick	Greenaway	17 January 1942
Catherine	Gurbutt	09 March 1970
Graham Peter	Hailey	30 March 1933
Arthur Stephen	Haywood	26 April 1913
Darryl Wayne	Hill	28 June 1942
David James	Hutchinson	10 September 1966
Raj	James	05 April 1943
Robert James	Miller	17 May 1969
Colin Stephen	Johanson	04 April 1979
Stephen James	Kidd	09 December 1955
Clive David	Lewis	04 May 1962
Ryan Stephen	Lodge	06 November 1969
Amanda	Lowry	28 October 1958
Catherine Susan	Maclean	23 June 1965
David John	Marshall	06 October 1928
Helen Beverley	Morris	20 January 1944
Nicholas Steven	Munro	08 July 1969
Paul John	Oakes	22 December 1934
Richard	Parkes	25 June 1936
Edwina	Parkinson	22 April 1938
Raj	Patel	31 January 1933
Stephen James	Smith	18 January 1965
Barbara	Pratt	22 August 1976
Duncan John	Pritchard	22 April 1936
Len Colin	Rawlinson	31 August 1964
Derek	Roberts	01 December 1976
Andrea Jane	Sanderson	20 August 1956
Elizabeth Mary	Sanderson	12 July 1973
Margaret Ann	Scanlon	26 May 1956
Anne Helen	Sheppard	17 October 1930
Michael Joseph	Sheward	23 April 1928
Duncan John	Smith	09 August 1945
Stephen Christopher	Steel	01 March 1920
Anne Helen	Townsend	27 April 1943
James Alexander	Turner	25 May 1958
Paul Eliot	Wainwright	18 June 1929
Stephen Michael	Watkinson	20 March 1950
Paul David	Webster	02 July 1920
Colin Stephen	Wesley	28 June 1943
Gordon James	Wilcock	18 July 1930
Elizabeth Catherine	Wilkinson	21 September 1963
Sharon	Wilson	25 June 1956

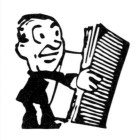

Smart Alec says
'For the really pedantic, it should be:

$$< \text{Now( )} - \text{Int}(18*365.25)$$

which takes account of leap years: but even then, there's 2000 to consider . . .

Very often in screening programmes we are interested in populations with upper and lower age limits, e.g. 18–55.

If we want to find those patients aged between 18 and 55, we must modify our expression to read as follows:

$$(< \text{Now( )} - \text{Int}(18*365.25)) \text{ And } (> \text{Now( )} - \text{Int}(55*365.25))$$

which, on a query run on 6 February 2002, produced the following results:

ForeNames	Surname	DateOfBirth
Tom	Jones	23 April 1954
Elaine	Smith	11 February 1961
Robert John	Peel	28 December 1952
Colin John	Adams	29 May 1957
Stephen John	Aggett	26 June 1964
Naomi Catherine	Armfield	27 March 1950
Sara Ann	Armstrong	09 August 1973
Sally Christine	Atkinson	13 February 1952
Heather	Bowker	25 November 1974
Alan Graham	Briggs	17 February 1955
Colin Stephen	Campbell	15 June 1968
Christine	Clough	14 April 1983
Margaret Ann	Corbett	04 July 1956
Robert Andrew	Crispin	19 November 1957
Stephen Ivor	Dexter	17 June 1975
Harold Anthony	Franks	05 February 1961
Elizabeth Catherine	Faulks	09 April 1972
John Paul	Gibbon	05 October 1948
Anna Elizabeth	Gillies	25 July 1951
Catherine	Gurbutt	09 March 1970
David James	Hutchinson	10 September 1966
Robert James	Miller	17 May 1969
Colin Stephen	Johanson	04 April 1979
Stephen James	Kidd	09 December 1955
Clive David	Lewis	04 May 1962

ForeNames	Surname	DateOfBirth
Ryan Stephen	Lodge	06 November 1969
Amanda	Lowry	28 October 1958
Catherine Susan	Maclean	23 June 1965
Nicholas Steven	Munro	08 July 1969
Stephen James	Smith	18 January 1965
Barbara	Pratt	22 August 1976
Len Colin	Rawlinson	31 August 1964
Derek	Roberts	01 December 1976
Andrea Jane	Sanderson	20 August 1956
Elizabeth Mary	Sanderson	12 July 1973
Margaret Ann	Scanlon	26 May 1956
James Alexander	Turner	25 May 1958
Stephen Michael	Watkinson	20 March 1950
Elizabeth Catherine	Wilkinson	21 September 1963
Sharon	Wilson	25 June 1956

All the patients listed were born between 6 February 1947 (55 years before the query was run) and 6 February 1984 (18 years before the query was run).

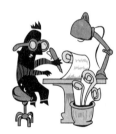

Over to you
Now try and run the following queries on this database:
- patients seeing Dr Howard on 23 February 2002
- patients under 18 who have seen Dr Shaw
- patients over 65 with 5 minute appointments.

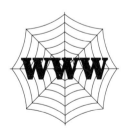

Web link
If you get stuck, try visiting the Chapter 4 section of the website to find query designs for these problems.

Reports

Reports provide a way of presenting data from tables or queries. They may be regarded as providing the same function for queries as forms for tables. We shall start with turning our query based upon the fields Start time (from Appointments), Duration (from Appointments), Surname (from Doctors) and Surname (from Patients) which was probably stored as 'Appointments Query1'.

Go to the main database window and select 'Reports' and then 'Create report by using wizard':

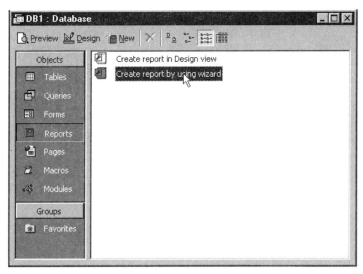

At the first dialog, select the query from the drop-down menu:

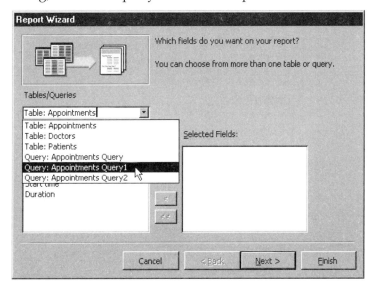

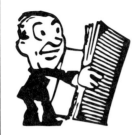

Smart Alec says
'You could construct the same result from its constitu-
ent tables by repeating the process we carried out when
we produced the original query.'

Select all the fields from the query by clicking on ≫:

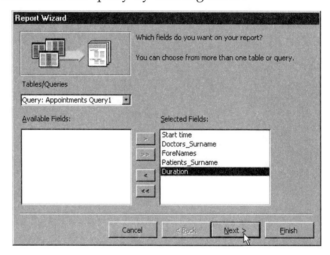

Click on Next >.

At the next dialog, we accept the option to order the information by
Appointments:

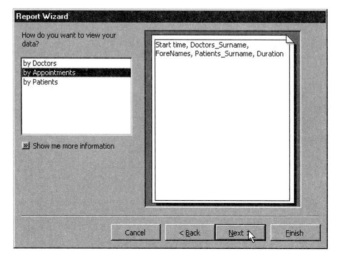

Click on Next >.

At the next dialog, we get the chance to add grouping levels. Let's keep it simple at this stage, shall we?

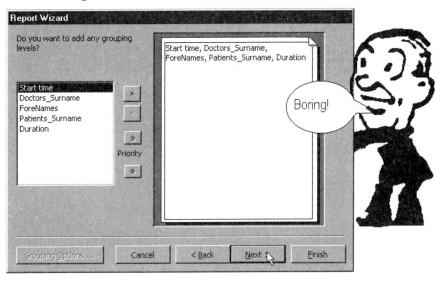

Click on Next >.

At the next dialog, we tell it to sort the data by Start time:

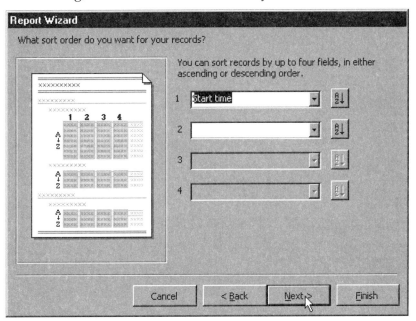

Click on Next >.

At the next dialog, choose a Tabular layout in Portrait orientation, since the report is relatively tall and narrow:

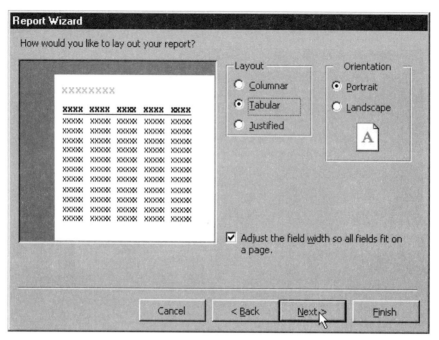

Click on Next >.

At the next of a seemingly endless stream of dialog boxes, choose a Formal style:

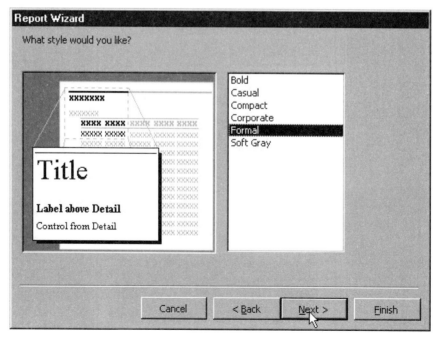

Click on Next >.

Finally, accept the name 'Appointments' and select the 'Preview the report' option:

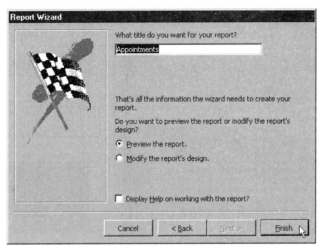

Click on Finish.

The finished report is shown in Print Preview mode:

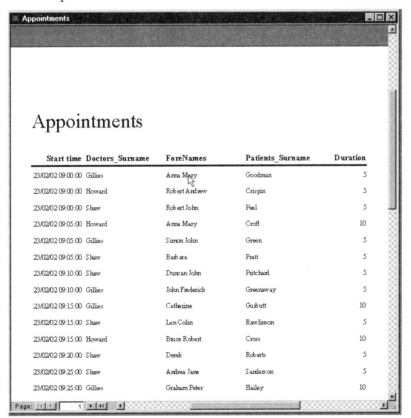

To see how this report is constructed, flip it over into Design view at the View icon 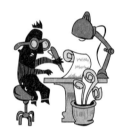 :

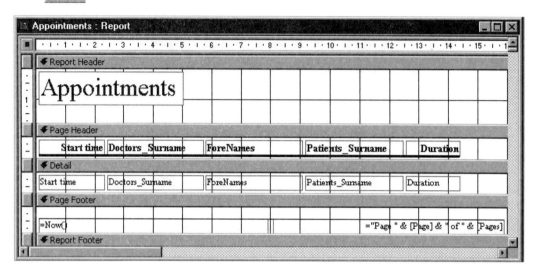

Over to you

You can create very differently ordered and looking reports using the different wizard options. Have a play with the following options and see what you create:

- ordering
- grouping level
- style
- layout.

By using the design view, you can change almost all the parameters. From your experience with forms, you should be able to change the header and footers to different colours. Try changing the background and font colours.

Now try and produce the following reports mirroring the queries suggested in the previous section:

- patients seeing Dr Howard on 23 February 2002
- patients under 18 who have seen Dr Shaw
- patients over 65 with 5 minute appointments.

Using an Access database with Word to produce recall letters

Supposing we want to recall all the children under the age of 11. We need to generate some nice letters to encourage them to come in and see us. We can write a letter in Word and then generate personalised letters using the data in our database.

Open Word and type the following letter.

The Health Centre,
The Square
PRESTON
PR1 2TQ

7 February 2002

To the parent/guardian of

Dear Parent/Guardian,

As part of our healthy children campaign, we are inviting all our children to visit the surgery to take advantage of the new meningitis vaccine during March.

We hope that we will see you there.

Yours faithfully

Dr A Gillies

Minimise the Word window at the bottom of the screen.

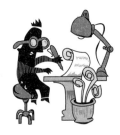

Over to you

Return to Access and write a query to select the children under 11. By now this should be within your capabilities. However, here are some hints:

1   Use the following fields from the Patients table:
    • ForeNames
    • Surname
    • Address1
    • Address2
    • PostalCode
    • DateOfBirth.
2   Call it 'Children'.
3   When finished the query should look like the one below.

Field:	ForeNames	Surname	Address1	Address2	PostalCode	DateOfBirth
Table:	Patients	Patients	Patients	Patients	Patients	Patients
Sort:						
Show:	☑	☑	☑	☑	☑	☐
Criteria:						>Now()-Int(11*365.25)
or:						

Run on 7 February 2002, it produced the following result:

ForeNames	Surname	Address1	Address2	Postal Code
Brian Antony	Jasper	451 Fylde Rd	Preston	PR1 2JO
Colin Stephen	Brown	23 Crompton St	Preston	
Anna Mary	Croft	11 London Rd	Wigan	
Lynn Helen	Lloyd	14 Lindley St	Lostock Hall, Preston	
Rachael Anna	Stapleton	15 Thanet Gro	Leigh	
Stephen John	Taylor	31 Dukes Meadow	Ingol, Preston	
Mark	Tomlinson	49 Greenford Clo	Orrell, Wigan	
Clive David	Watts	13 Greyfriars	Ashton In Makerfield, Wigan	

Now minimise the Access window, and return to Word.
   Select the Mail Merge option from the <u>T</u>ools menu.

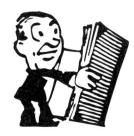

Smart Alec says

'If you can't find Mail Merge on your Tools menu, it's because Word has taken it away as it's not been used. Click on the double chevron at the bottom of the menu to reveal all the options. Can't stand it when computers try to be smart . . .'

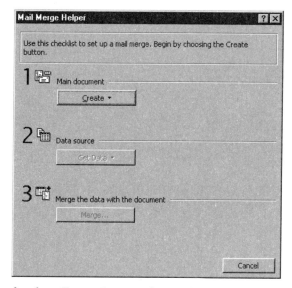

Click on <u>C</u>reate and select Form <u>L</u>etters from the menu:

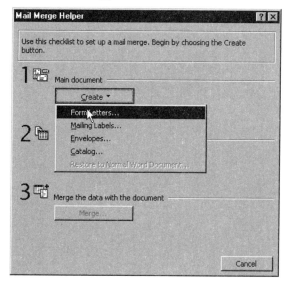

You have already created the basis of your letter, so select Active Window:

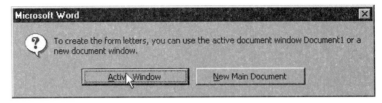

At the next dialog, select Open Data Source from the Get Data menu:

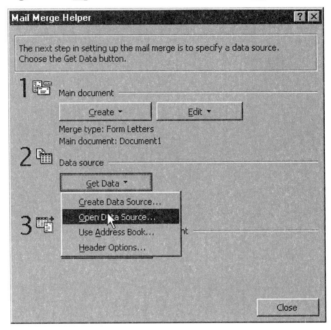

At the Open dialog, select MS Access Databases as the file type, and then the database containing the patient data (mine is saved as 'db1'), and click on the Queries tab:

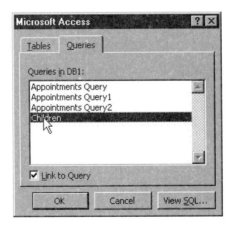

Select the Children query.
Click on OK.

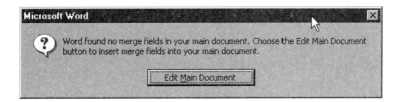

Now use the Insert Merge field menu to add merge fields to your letter:

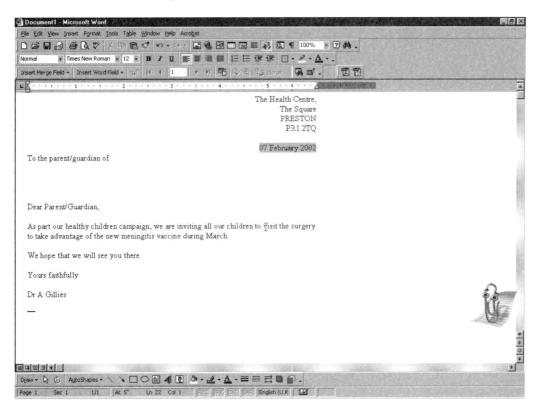

Until it looks like the one below:

The Health Centre,
The Square
PRESTON
PR1 2TQ

7 February 2002

To the parent/guardian of

«ForeNames» «Surname»,
«Address1»
«Address2»
«PostalCode»

Dear Parent/Guardian,

As part our healthy children campaign, we are inviting all our children to visit the surgery to take advantage of the new meningitis vaccine during March.

We hope that we will see you there.

Yours faithfully

Dr A Gillies

Now if we merge the letter and the query we should produce a letter for each patient:

The Health Centre,
The Square
PRESTON
PR1 2TQ

7 February 2002

To the parent/guardian of

Brian Antony Jasper,
451 Fylde Rd
Preston
PR1 2JO

Dear Parent/Guardian,

As part our healthy children campaign, we are inviting all our children to visit the surgery to take advantage of the new meningitis vaccine during March.

We hope that we will see you there.

Yours faithfully

Dr A Gillies

The Health Centre,
The Square
PRESTON
PR1 2TQ

7 February 2002

To the parent/guardian of

Colin Stephen Brown,
23 Crompton St
Preston

Dear Parent/Guardian,

The Health Centre,
The Square
PRESTON
PR1 2TQ

7 February 2002

To the parent/guardian of

Anna Mary Croft,
11 London Rd
Wigan

Dear Parent/Guardian,

The Health Centre,
The Square
PRESTON
PR1 2TQ

7 February 2002

To the parent/guardian of

Lynn Helen Lloyd,
14 Lindley St
Lostock Hall, Preston

Dear Parent/Guardian,

The Health Centre,
The Square
PRESTON
PR1 2TQ

7 February 2002

To the parent/guardian of

Rachael Anna Stapleton,
15 Thanet Gro
Leigh

Dear Parent/Guardian,

The Health Centre,
The Square
PRESTON
PR1 2TQ

7 February 2002

To the parent/guardian of

Stephen John Taylor,
31 Dukes Meadow
Ingol, Preston

Dear Parent/Guardian,

The Health Centre,
The Square
PRESTON
PR1 2TQ

7 February 2002

To the parent/guardian of

Mark Tomlinson,
49 Greenford Clo
Orrell, Wigan

Dear Parent/Guardian,

The Health Centre,
The Square
PRESTON
PR1 2TQ

7 February 2002

To the parent/guardian of

Clive David Watts,
13 Greyfriars
Ashton In Makerfield, Wigan

Dear Parent/Guardian,

5

Where do we go to from here?

Introduction

The problem with Access is that it is a very versatile and therefore quite a complex application. We have barely scraped the surface of what it can do. Therefore the purpose of this chapter is to point you in the direction of resources which can take you further on and further in . . .

The help facility

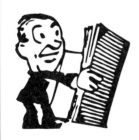

Smart Alec says
'That damned paper clip isn't nearly as good-looking as me, but actually once you know a bit, then the help facility can be actually helpful.'

If you don't like the paper clip, then you can disable it and use the Help menu instead.

For example, we didn't deal with headers and footers on forms. Supposing you want to find out more?

From the Help menu, select Microsoft Access Help. It provides a whole range of ways to find help.

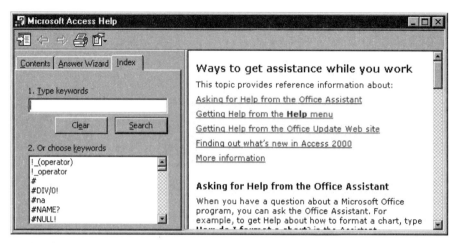

You can look up things in the contents, question the answer wizard or give the index keywords. We'll give the index the keyword 'header'.

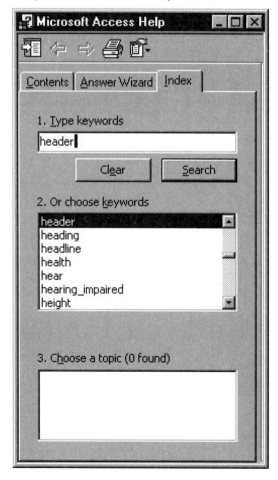

Then click on Search:

The fourth topic is 'Add or remove a form header and footer'.

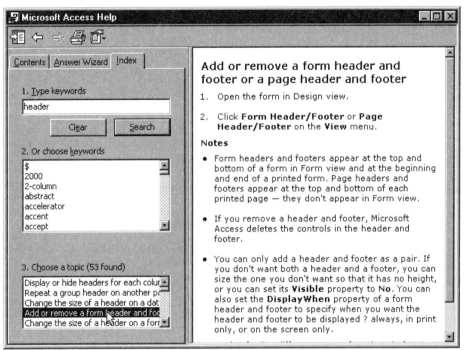

The explanation says:

---

1 Open the form in Design view.
2 Click **Form Header/Footer** or **Page Header/Footer** on the **View** menu.

Notes

- Form headers and footers appear at the top and bottom of a form in Form view and at the beginning and end of a printed form. Page headers and footers appear at the top and bottom of each printed page – they don't appear in Form view.
- If you remove a header and footer, Microsoft Access deletes the controls in the header and footer.
- You can only add a header and footer as a pair. If you don't want both a header and a footer, you can size the one you don't want so that it has no height, or you can set its **Visible** property to **No**. You can also set the DisplayWhen property of a form header and footer to specify when you want the header and footer to be displayed always, in print only, or on the screen only.

Books

Sometimes the help facility just isn't enough. Fortunately, there are many books out there.

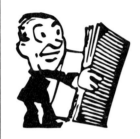

Smart Alec says
'OK, smarty pants, so why did you write this one?'

'Because I don't know one written for healthcare workers which is straightforward and not full of examples of second-hand car salesmen from Idaho.'

'Ooh! Pardon me for asking . . . !'

This book seeks to provide a basic and readable beginner's guide. Some of the recent more technical books available for purchase online on Access 2000 include:

1   Forte S (1999) *Microsoft Access 2000 Development: Unleashed.* Sams, Indianapolis, IN.
2   Callahan E (1999) *Microsoft Access 2000 Visual Basic for Applications.* CD-ROM. Microsoft Press International, Seattle, WA.
3   Prague CN and Irwin MR (1999) *Microsoft Access 2000 Bible.* Hungry Minds Inc, New York.
4   Dobson R (2000) *Professional Sql Server Development with Access 2000.* Wrox Press Ltd.
5   Course Technology (ed.) (2000) *Data-driven Web Sites with Microsoft Access 2000.* Thomson Learning, Florence KY.
6   Oxford K (2000) *New Perspectives on Microsoft Access 2000 with VBA – Advanced.* Thomson Learning, Florence KY.

And, for any visiting Spanish doctors or nurses:

• Dario Angel Gonzalez *et al.* (1999) *MS Office 2000, 4 Libros en 1 con CD-ROM: Manuales Users, en Espanol.* MP Ediciones SA.

In all, Amazon listed 97 titles relating to Access 2000 alone. I do not endorse them, I merely point out their existence!

Online resources

There are a wealth of online resources. As these change frequently, I shan't list them here, but refer you instead to the website.

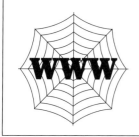

Web link
From the Chapter 5 section of the website accompanying this book you can access a range of online resources.

Courses

The NHS is currently investing a significant level of resource in basic IT training linked to the ECDL. You should be able to access this training at no cost to yourself if you are an NHS staff member.

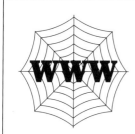

Web link
In the Chapter 5 section of the website accompanying this book you will find links to the ECDL website, which tells you about the ECDL, and the NHSIA website, which tells you what the NHS is doing about it nationally.

NHS contacts

There is a range of people employed to help you develop your skills. Try contacting your local Education, Training and Development Lead or your local LIS co-ordinator. I will publish contact details via the website where available.

Appendix: Description of the database used in Chapter 4

The three tables used in the database application are populated as follows.

Doctors

GMCNumber	Forenames	Surname	Extension	Mobile
1234567	Alan	Gillies	2135	(0794) 1826542
345789	John	Howard	2137	(0794) 6753212
432564	Nicola	Shaw	2134	(0780) 3421567

Patients

NHSNumber	ForeNames	Surname	Address1	Address2	Postal Code	Phone Number	DateOfBirth	Title
191224	Emma Jane	Abbott	8 Church Av	Penwortham, Preston			07 June 1932	Mr
145897	Colin John	Adams	45a Fylde Rd	Ashton On Ribble, Preston		223413	29 May 1957	Mr
175181	Stephen John	Aggett	3 Hesketh Meadow La	Lowton, Warrington		345123	26 June 1964	Mr
227835	Naomi Catherine	Armfield	31 Parklands Dv	Fulwood, Preston		456798	27 March 1950	Mrs
910806	Sara Ann	Armstrong	122 Powys Rd	Fulwood, Preston		564342	09 August 1973	Ms
268696	Sally Christine	Atkinson	10 Eldon St	Fulwood, Preston		567891	13 February 1952	Mrs
304578	Beverley Ann	Banks	45 Moss La	Leyland		890231	25 April 1915	Mrs
533930	Jennifer Susan	Blaylock	70 Preston Rd	Standish, Wigan		675412	02 August 1916	Mrs
177400	Emma Susan	Bowers	104 Watling St Rd	Fulwood, Preston			04 January 1932	Mr
708307	Heather	Bowker	14 Stour Ldg	Fulwood, Preston			25 November 1974	Ms
463426	Alan Graham	Briggs	52 Station Rd	Bamber Bridge, Preston		342765	17 February 1955	Mr
635458	Colin Stephen	Brown	23 Crompton St	Preston		987634	03 March 2001	Mr
285477	Kate Anne	Burrows	170 Bolton Rd	Ashton-In-Makerfield, Wigan		323454	19 July 1914	Mrs
143982	Colin Stephen	Campbell	28 Railway Lane	Walton Le Dale, Preston		123453	15 June 1968	Mr
575029	Clive Stephen	Chambers	12 Station Rd	Croston, LEYLAND	PR6 6DF	678543	20 May 1916	Mr
196027	Rachel Susan	Charlton	539 Warrington Rd	Ince, Wigan			03 October 1921	Mrs
315738	Michael John	Christie	23 Leeds Rd	Ashton In Makerfield, Wigan			24 September 1919	Mr
963024	Jennifer Cathryn	Clayton	1A Beckett Ct	Preston			24 May 1919	Mrs
154915	Christine	Clough	212 Brook St	Ribbleton, Preston			14 April 1983	Mrs
785289	Margaret Ann	Corbett	39 Wigan Rd	Orrell, Wigan			04 July 1956	Dr
450404	Robert Andrew	Crispin	12 Parbold Rd	Standish, Wigan			19 November 1957	Mr
436771	Anna Mary	Croft	11 London Rd	Wigan			07 September 2000	Ms
203997	Bruce Robert	Cross	21 Station Rd	Leigh			06 November 1919	Mr
341884	David John	Davies	28 Deepdale RD	Preston			17 January 1929	Mr
556900	Imogen	Davis	17 Church Brow	Walton Le Dale, Preston			18 June 1925	Ms
113679	Christine	Deighton	122 Powys Rd	Lea, Preston	PR3 1ER	136257	19 March 1940	Ms
202093	Stephen Ivor	Dexter	47 Newton Road	Ashton In Makerfield, Wigan			17 June 1975	Mr

Number	First Name	Surname	Address	Town	Postcode	Phone	Date	Title
568797	Mary Anne	Dobbs	32 Ribble Ave	Penwortham, Preston			14 July 1923	Mrs
104475	Lesley	Donaldson	5 Canal lane	Walton Le Dale, Preston	PR6 1VC	208149	30 September 1917	Mr
197099	Sara-Jane	Edwards	325 Eaves La	Chorley			26 June 1917	Mr
644100	Tracy Emma	Elliot	4 Margaret St	Wigan	WN3 7UH		04 September 1914	Ms
800340	Ronald James	Evans	10 Fairhaven Rd	Penwortham, Preston			03 June 1942	Mr
471498	Nigel Henry	Evans	56a Helvellyn Rd	Wigan			14 November 1945	Mr
150244	Elizabeth Catherine	Faulks	18 Whitegate Lane	Chorley			09 April 1972	Ms
815502	Paul David	Francis	23 Brook St	Preston			12 April 1944	Mr
683516	Harold Anthony	Franks	3 Lonmore	Walton Le Dale, Preston			05 February 1961	Mr
458053	Henry Cecil	Freeman	23 Ribble Ave	Ribbleton, Preston			17 November 1936	Mr
257526	John Paul	Gibbon	82 St. Thomas Rd	Preston	PR1 4DF	564532	05 October 1948	Mr
474924	Roger Brian	Gill	28 Salisbury St	Southport			12 March 1927	Mr
519576	Malcolm	Gillett	36 Seven Stars Rd	Leyland	PR6 6DF	433211	10 September 1922	Mr
755475	Anna Elizabeth	Gillies	22 Darvel Av	Ashton In Makerfield, Wigan			25 July 1951	Ms
651592	Samuel Stephen	Goodacre	82 Holden Rd	Leigh			31 August 1928	Mr
913882	Anna Mary	Goodman	16 Wilmot Rd	Leigh,			02 July 1942	Mrs
184619	Simon John	Green	6 Craigflower Ct	Bamber Bridge, Preston	PR6 3DC	332245	23 June 1928	Mr
515652	John Frederick	Greenaway	52 Liverpool Rd	Penwortham, Preston			17 January 1942	Rev
686403	Catherine	Gurbutt	Honeycomb House Pauls Sq	Preston			09 March 1970	Ms
941423	Graham Peter	Hailey	234 Blackpool Rd	Lea, Preston			30 March 1933	Mr
399385	Arthur Stephen	Haywood	187 Whitegate Drive	Blackpool			26 April 1913	Mr
635473	Darryl Wayne	Hill	12 Royden Rd	Billinge, Wigan			28 June 1942	Mr
518030	David James	Hutchinson	4 Kirkstall Clo	Chorley			10 September 1966	Mr
847938	Raj	James	112 London Rd	Walton Le Dale, Preston			05 April 1943	Mr
102485	Brian Antony	Jasper	451 Fylde Rd	Preston	PR1 2JO	331777	13 December 1997	Mr
257573	Colin Stephen	Johanson	20 Stanley Croft	Woodplumpton, Preston			04 April 1979	Mr
987654	Tom	Jones	21 Lowndes St	Preston	PR1 7XE	555432	23 April 1954	Mr
737807	Stephen James	Kidd	114 Threefields	Ingol, Preston			09 December 1955	Mr
891332	Clive David	Lewis	23 Hoole Road	New Longton, Preston			04 May 1962	Mr
303023	Lynn Helen	Lloyd	14 Lindley St	Lostock Hall, Preston			30 December 1991	Ms
535961	Ryan Stephen	Lodge	27 Leigh Lane	Ashton-In-Makerfield, Wigan			06 November 1969	Mr

Patients (cont.)

NHSNumber	ForeNames	Surname	Address1	Address2	Postal Code	Phone Number	DateOfBirth	Title
255138	Amanda	Lowry	23 Newton Rd	Ashton In Makerfield, Wigan			28 October 1958	Ms
226180	Catherine Susan	Maclean	12Lt Hoole Lane	Lowton, Warrington			23 June 1965	Mrs
804899	David John	Marshall	10 Stour Ldg	Southport			06 October 1928	Mr
258471	Robert James	Miller	7 Bannister Brook Ho Pearfield	LEYLAND			17 May 1969	Mr
529112	Helen Beverley	Morris	22 Church Av	Billinge, Wigan			20 January 1944	Mrs
454240	Nicholas Steven	Munro	57 Wyre Ave	Penwortham, Preston			08 July 1969	Mr
600164	Paul John	Oakes	24 Marston Moor	Fulwood, Preston			22 December 1934	Mr
859363	Richard	Parkes	312 Garstang Road	Fulwood, Preston			25 June 1936	Mr
240581	Edwina	Parkinson	23 Hoole Road	Penwortham, Preston			22 April 1938	Ms
866664	Raj	Patel	5a Charlesway Ct Lea Rd	Lea, Preston			31 January 1933	Mr
134045	Robert John	Peel	22 Darvel Av	Ashton In Makerfield, Wigan	WN4 3KB	705558	28 December 1952	Mr
207945	Barbara	Pratt	103 Moor Rd	Croston, LEYLAND			22 August 1976	Ms
601289	Duncan John	Pritchard	23a Hough lane	LEYLAND			22 April 1936	Mr
653597	Len Colin	Rawlinson	11 Hill Road Sth	Preston			31 August 1964	Mr
331559	Derek	Roberts	99 Cunliffe Rd	Blackpool			01 December 1976	Mr
261864	Andrea Jane	Sanderson	20 Bussell Rd	Penwortham, Preston			20 August 1956	Mr
836778	Elizabeth Mary	Sanderson	10 Wilmot Rd	Ribbleton, Preston			12 July 1973	Mr
922467	Margaret Ann	Scanlon	112 London Rd	LEYLAND			26 May 1956	Ms
328604	Anne Helen	Sheppard	14 Eldon St	Preston			17 October 1930	Mrs
418577	Michael Joseph	Sheward	7 Riversmeade	Leigh,			23 April 1928	Mr
112452	Elaine	Smith	11 Church Side	New Longton, Preston	PR6 1BN	214563	11 February 1961	Ms
756764	Stephen James	Smith	789 Blackpool Rd	Lea, Preston			18 January 1965	Mr
976539	Duncan John	Smith	904 Blackpool Rd	Lea, Preston			09 August 1945	Mr
718251	Rachael Anna	Stapleton	15 Thanet Gro	Leigh, Wigan			20 June 1992	Ms
238839	Stephen	Steel	57 Mersey Ave				01 March 1920	Mr
916506	Christopher Stephen John	Taylor	31 Dukes Meadow	Ingol, Preston			26 February 1993	Mr

ID	Surname	First names	Address	Area	Postcode	Ref	Date	Title
531967	Tomlinson	Mark	49 Greenford Clo	Orrell, Wigan			08 January 1992	Mr
346147	Townsend	Anne Helen	51 Canal lane	Ingol, Preston			27 April 1943	Mrs
645905	Turner	James Alexander	17 Hill Road Sth	Penwortham, Preston			25 May 1958	Mr
300525	Wainwright	Paul Eliot	28 Railway St	Chorley	PR7 5FG	743256	18 June 1929	Mr
857151	Watkinson	Stephen Michael	9 Hawkshead Rd	Ribbleton, Preston			20 March 1950	Mr
942507	Watts	Clive David	13 Greyfriars	Ashton In Makerfield, Wigan			06 November 1997	Mr
703121	Webster	Paul David	15 Lowesby Clo	Walton Le Dale, Preston			02 July 1920	Mr
457195	Wesley	Colin Stephen	141 Newton Road	Lostock Hall, Preston			28 June 1943	Mr
542823	West	Peter Graham	23 Newton Rd	Lea, Preston			05 June 1990	Mr
748395	Wilcock	Gordon James	131 Slater La	Preston			18 July 1930	Mr
282858	Wilkinson	Elizabeth Catherine	36 Moss La	LEYLAND			21 September 1963	Ms
379709	Wilson	Simon John	1 Kirkland Pl	Ashton On Ribble, Preston			09 June 1984	Mr
331145	Wilson	Sharon	39 Back Lane	Fulwood, Preston			25 June 1956	Ms

Appointments

AppointmentID	NHSNumber	GMCNumber	Start time		Duration
1	450404	345789	23/02/02	09:00:00	5
2	436771	345789	23/02/02	09:05:00	10
3	203997	345789	23/02/02	09:15:00	10
4	341884	345789	23/02/02	09:25:00	10
5	556900	345789	23/02/02	09:35:00	10
6	113679	345789	23/02/02	09:45:00	10
7	202093	345789	23/02/02	09:55:00	10
8	568797	345789	23/02/02	10:05:00	10
9	104475	345789	23/02/02	10:15:00	10
10	197099	345789	23/02/02	10:25:00	10
11	644100	345789	23/02/02	10:35:00	15
12	800340	345789	23/02/02	10:50:00	10
13	471498	345789	24/02/02	09:00:00	10
14	150244	345789	24/02/02	09:10:00	10
15	815502	345789	24/02/02	09:20:00	10
16	683516	345789	24/02/02	09:30:00	10
17	458053	345789	24/02/02	09:40:00	10
18	257526	345789	24/02/02	09:50:00	10
19	474924	345789	24/02/02	10:00:00	15
20	519576	345789	24/02/02	10:15:00	5
21	755475	345789	24/02/02	10:20:00	5
22	651592	345789	24/02/02	10:25:00	5
23	913882	1234567	23/02/02	09:00:00	5
24	184619	1234567	23/02/02	09:05:00	5
25	515652	1234567	23/02/02	09:10:00	5
26	686403	1234567	23/02/02	09:15:00	10
27	941423	1234567	23/02/02	09:25:00	10
28	399385	1234567	23/02/02	09:35:00	10
29	635473	1234567	23/02/02	09:45:00	10
30	518030	1234567	23/02/02	09:55:00	10
31	847938	1234567	23/02/02	10:05:00	10
32	102485	1234567	23/02/02	10:15:00	10
33	257573	1234567	23/02/02	10:25:00	10
34	737807	1234567	23/02/02	10:35:00	10
35	891332	1234567	23/02/02	10:45:00	15
36	303023	1234567	24/02/02	09:00:00	10
37	535961	1234567	24/02/02	09:10:00	10
38	255138	1234567	24/02/02	09:20:00	10
39	226180	1234567	24/02/02	09:30:00	10
40	804899	1234567	24/02/02	09:40:00	10
41	258471	1234567	24/02/02	09:50:00	10

Appointments (cont.)

AppointmentID	NHSNumber	GMCNumber	Start time		Duration
42	529112	1234567	24/02/02	10:00:00	5
43	454240	1234567	24/02/02	10:05:00	5
44	600164	1234567	24/02/02	10:10:00	5
45	859363	1234567	24/02/02	10:15:00	15
46	240581	1234567	24/02/02	10:30:00	15
47	866664	1234567	24/02/02	10:45:00	15
48	134045	432564	23/02/02	09:00:00	5
49	207945	432564	23/02/02	09:05:00	5
50	601289	432564	23/02/02	09:10:00	5
51	653597	432564	23/02/02	09:15:00	5
52	331559	432564	23/02/02	09:20:00	5
53	261864	432564	23/02/02	09:25:00	5
54	836778	432564	23/02/02	09:30:00	5
55	922467	432564	23/02/02	09:35:00	5
56	328604	432564	23/02/02	09:40:00	5
57	418577	432564	23/02/02	09:45:00	5
58	756764	432564	23/02/02	09:50:00	5
59	976539	432564	23/02/02	09:55:00	5
60	112452	432564	23/02/02	10:00:00	10
61	718251	432564	23/02/02	10:10:00	10
62	238839	432564	23/02/02	10:20:00	10
63	916506	432564	23/02/02	10:30:00	10
64	531967	432564	23/02/02	10:40:00	10
65	346147	432564	23/02/02	10:50:00	10
66	645905	432564	24/02/02	09:00:00	10
67	300525	432564	24/02/02	09:10:00	10
68	857151	432564	24/02/02	09:20:00	10
69	942507	432564	24/02/02	09:30:00	10
70	703121	432564	24/02/02	09:40:00	10
71	457195	432564	24/02/02	09:50:00	10
72	542823	432564	24/02/02	10:00:00	15
73	748395	432564	24/02/02	10:15:00	15
74	282858	432564	24/02/02	10:30:00	15
75	379709	432564	24/02/02	10:45:00	15
76	331145	432564	24/02/02	11:00:00	20

Index